MODELS OF ANAEROBIC INFECTION

NEW PERSPECTIVES IN CLINICAL MICROBIOLOGY

Brumfitt W, ed Hamilton-Miller JMT, assist. ed: New perspectives in clinical micro-
biology. 1978. ISBN 90-247-2074-5
Tyrrell DAJ, ed: Aspects of slow and persistent virus infections. 1979.
ISBN 90-247-2281-0
Brumfitt W, Curcio L, Silvestri L, eds: Combined antimicrobial therapy. 1979.
ISBN 90-247-2280-2
van Furth R, ed: Developments in antibiotic treatment of respiratory infections. 1981.
ISBN 90-247-2493-7
van Furth R, ed: Evaluation and management of hospital infections. 1982.
ISBN 90-247-2754-5
Kuwahara S, Pierce NF, eds: Advances in research on cholera and related diarrheas 1.
1983. ISBN 0-89838-592-X
Ristic M, Ambroise-Thomas P, Kreier J, eds: Malaria and babesiosis: Research findings
and control measures. 1984. ISBN 0-89838-675-6
Kuwahara S, Pierce NF, eds: Advances in research on cholera and related diarrheas 2.
1984. ISBN 0-89838-680-2
Takeda Y: Bacterial diarrheal diseases. 1984. ISBN 0-89838-681-0
Hill MJ, Borriello SP, Hardie JM, Hudson MJ, Lysons RJ, Tabaqchali S, eds: Models
of anaerobic infection.
1984. ISBN 0-89838-688-8

MODELS OF ANAEROBIC INFECTION

Proceedings of the third Anaerobe Discussion Group Symposium held at Churchill College, University of Cambridge, July 30–31, 1983, followed by the abstracts of the first meeting of the Society for Intestinal Microbial Ecology and Disease, Boston, November 1983

edited by the steering committee of the Anaerobe Discussion Group

editor in chief:
M.J. HILL

members:
S.P. BORRIELLO, J.M. HARDIE, M.J. HUDSON, R.J. LYSONS, S. TABAQCHALI

1984 **MARTINUS NIJHOFF PUBLISHERS**
a member of the KLUWER ACADEMIC PUBLISHERS GROUP
DORDRECHT / BOSTON / LANCASTER

Distributors

for the United States and Canada: Kluwer Academic Publishers, 190 Old Derby Street, Hingham, MA 02043, USA
for the UK and Ireland: Kluwer Academic Publishers, MTP Press Limited, Falcon House, Queen Square, Lancaster LA1 1RN, England
for all other countries: Kluwer Academic Publishers Group, Distribution Center, P.O. Box 322, 3300 AH Dordrecht, The Netherlands

Library of Congress Cataloging in Publication Data

ISBN 0-89838-688-8 (this volume)

Copyright

PRINTED IN THE NETHERLANDS

PREFACE

The ADG held its first International Symposium at Churchill College,
Cambridge, in July 1979. The second symposium was also held at Churchill
College on 30-31 July, 1981, and this, the third, took place at the same
college on 30-31 July, 1983.

The meeting was structured in a format which we hoped would appeal to
the full range of our membership. The philosophy of the ADG is that
medical microbiologists, veterinarians, toxicologists and dental
bacteriologists have much to learn from each other and can best be
achieved by bringing these various disciplines together frequently and
in informal surroundings. Again the symposium was very generously
sponsored by May and Baker Limited who met all costs of the meeting and
entertained us splendidly. David Jackson and Donald Bedford were responsible for coordinating with the ADG on behalf of May and Baker and,
as usual, gave us their full cooperation.

This book contains the full-length papers, followed by the posters
presented at the meeting.

This book also serves as a vehicle for the abstracts of the first meeting
of the Society for Intestinal Microbial Ecology and Disease, SIMED, held
in Boston, Massachusetts. An introduction to this new society by its
President, Sydney M. Finegold, M.D., precedes the abstracts.

M.J. Hill

VI

CONTENTS

LIST OF CONTRIBUTORS

Barer, M.R.
Department of Medical Microbiology, London School of Hygiene and Tropical Medicine, Keppel Street (Gower St.), London, WC1E 7HT.

Borriello, S.P.
Division of Communicable Diseases, Clinical Research Centre, Watford Road, Harrow, Middlesex, HA1 3UJ.

Burman, L.G.
Lasarattet, Klt Bakt Lab., 721 89 Veastaras, Sweden.

Carman, R.J.
Animal Unit, Charing Cross Hospital Medical School, St. Dunstan's Road, London, W6 8RP.

Carlsson, J.
Department of Endodontics, School of Dentistry, University of Umeå, Umeå 6, Sweden.

Connolly, Janet C.
Department of Medical Microbiology, St. Bartholomew's Hospital Medical College, London, EC1.

Drasar, B.S.
Department of Medical Microbiology, London School of Hygiene and Tropical Medicine, Keppel Street (Gower St.), London, WC1 7HT.

Ellwood, D.C.
PHLS Centre for Applied Microbiology and Research, Pathogenic Microbes Research Laboratory, Porton Down, Salisbury, Wiltshire, SP4 0JG.

Gemmel, C.G.
University of Glasgow, Bacteriology Department, Royal Infirmary, Glasgow, G4 0SF.

Giugliano, L.G.
Department of Medical Microbiology, London School of Hygiene and Tropical Medicine, Keppel Street (Gower St.), London, WC1E 7HT.

Guggenheim, B., Gmur, R. and Wyss, C.
University of Zürich, Zahnärzliches Institut, Plattenstrasse 11, CH-8028, Zürich.

Hill, M.J.
PHLS Centre for Applied Microbiology and Research, Bacterial Metabolism Research Laboratory, Porton Down, Salisbury, Wiltshire, SP4 0JG.

Hine, Paul M.
Department of Bacteriology R&D, The Wellcome Research Laboratories, Langley Court, Beckenham, Kent, BR3 3BS.

Hobson, P.N.
The Rowett Research Institute, Microbial Biochemistry Department, Greenburn Road, Bucksburn, Aberdeen, AB2 9SB.

Holm, S.E.
Lasarattet, KLT Bakt Lab., 721 89 Veastaras, Sweden.

Hungate, R.E.	University of California, Department of Bacteriology, Davis California 95616, USA.
Ingham, H.R.	Department of Microbiology, Institute of Pathology, General Hospital, Westgate Road, Newcastle-Upon-Tyne, NE4 6BE.
Jones, G.R.	University of Glasgow, Bacteriology Department, Royal Infirmary, Glasgow, G4 0SF.
Kelly, M.J.	Department of Surgery, Southmead General Hospital, Westbury-on-Trym, Bristol, BS10 5NB.
Lysons, R.J.	ARC Institute for Research on Animal Diseases, Compton, Nr. Newbury, Berkshire, RG16 0NN.
McDermid, Ann S.	PHLS Centre for Applied Microbiology and Research, Pathogenic Microbes Research Laboratory, Porton Down, Salisbury, Wiltshire, SP4 0JG.
McKee, Ailsa S.	PHLS Centre for Applied Microbiology and Research, Pathogenic Microbes Research Laboratory, Porton Down, Salisbury, Wiltshire, SP4 0JG.
McNaught, R.	University of Glasgow, Bacteriology Department, Royal Infirmary, Glasgow, G4 0SF.
Mann, G.F.	Department of Medical Microbiology, London School of Hygiene and Tropical Medicine, Keppel Street (Gower St.), London, WC1E 7HT.
Marsh, P.D.	PHLS Centre for Applied Microbiology and Research, Pathogenic Microbes Research Laboratory, Porton Down, Salisbury, Wiltshire, SP4 0JG.
Nord, C.E. and Lahnborg, G.	The National Bacteriological Laboratory, S-105 21 Stockholm, Sweden.
Price, A.	Department of Histopathology, Northwick Park Hospital and Clinical Research Centre, Watford Road, Harrow, Middlesex, HA1 3UJ.
Rowland, I.R.	British Industrial Biological Research Association, Woodmansterne Road, Carshalton, Surrey, SM5 4DS.
Sisson, Penelope R.	Department of Microbiology, Institute of Pathology, General Hospital, Westgate Road, Newcastle-Upon-Tyne, NE4 6BE.
Sundqvist, G.	Department of Endodontics, School of Dentistry, University of Umeå, Umeå 6, Sweden.
Tabaqchali, Soad	Department of Medical Microbiology, St. Bartholomew's Hospital Medical College, London, EC1.

Thore, M.

Lasarattet, KLT Bakt Lab., 721 89 Veastaras, Sweden.

Walker, P.D.

Department of Bacteriology R&D, The Wellcome Research Laboratories, Langley Court, Beckenham, Kent, BR3 3BS.

Wyss, C.

University of Zurich, Zahnärzliches Institut, Plattenstrasse 11, CH-8028 Zürich.

INTRODUCTION TO THE ANAEROBIC DISCUSSION GROUP

The Anaerobe Discussion Group (ADG) was formed in 1975 when 16
people working on various aspects of anaerobe bacteriology met at
the Central Public Health Laboratory, London, to exchange
information and ideas. The initial group included people interested
in human infection, the human gut, dental bacteriology, veterinary
bacteriology and toxicology and it quickly became apparent that the
various subgroups could benefit greatly from each others expertise,
and so we have attempted to maintain this mix of interests and,
where possible, to extend it. The aim of the group is to raise the
technical standards of anaerobic bacteriology to the maximum and to
raise the general awareness of the function of anaerobic bacteria in
health and disease. It holds 3 or 4 meetings each year, usually on
Tuesday afternoons in one of the London Medical Schools, and has had
26 meetings to date.

The ADG has no formal constitution or membership but has a
mailing list of more than 250 and the average attendance at meetings
during the last few years has been 50-60. It is run by a "steering
committee" of 6 persons, namely Peter Borriello (CRC, Northwick Park
Hospital), Jeremy Hardie (London Hospital Dental School), Michael
Hill (CAMR) Michael Hudson (CAMR), Richard Lysons (ARC, Compton) and
Soad Tabaqchali (St.Bartholomews Hospital). Most of the people on
the mailing list and who attend meetings live in the London area but
the number from further afield (particularly Scotland) increases
annually. The group particularly welcomes people who are new to the
field of anaerobic bacteriology, whether from Hospitals, Dental
Schools, Veterinary institutes or industry and people who wish to be
added to the mailing list should write to any of the steering
committee members.

A guinea-pig model demonstrating synergy between Escherichia coli
and Bacteroides fragilis in infected surgical wounds.

M.J. Kelly

SUMMARY

Known numbers of standard NCTC strain of E. coli and B. fragilis
were inoculated separately and together into surgical incisions in
guinea-pigs. Histological and quantitative bacteriological proof is
presented that pathogenic synergy occurred in vivo when doses of
each organism that were separately subinfective were combined into
an aerobe-anaerobe mixture. A further series of experiments showed
that the amounts and ratio of the two organisms, in the challenge
inocula were critical, and the resultant pus contained equal numbers
of both the aerobic and anaerobic organism, despite their having
been disparate in the challenge inocula.

INTRODUCTION

A series of clinical trials at Addenbrooke's Hospital, Cambridge
indicated that wounds from which a mixed growth of aerobes and
anaerobes could be cultured carried a 71% rate of subsequent
clinical infection (1). An animal model was developed to test the
hypothesis of aerobe-anaerobe synergy (2).

ORGANISMS

Organisms representative of the commonest aerobes and anaerobes
grown above were Escherichia coli strain NCTC9434 and Bacteroides
fragilis NCTC9343. Separate 0.5 ml portions from 100 ml of culture
of each organism were frozen, and uniformity was secured by using
dilutions of these portions after thawing for all the experiments.

ANIMAL MODEL

Under neuroleptanalgesia (3) four measured 2 cm wounds were made
in the suprascapular area of adult female albino guinea-pigs. Each
wound was inoculated with 0.1 ml of a dilution of bacterial
suspension containing one or both organisms. The incisions were
closed with Michel clips (not stitches) and covered with a
vapour-permeable "Op-Site" dressing (4). At sacrifice, on the 7th
day, standard measured blocks of tissue were excised each including
a test wound and homogenised in a Colworth Stomacher machine (5).
Bacterial viable counts were performed on the centrifuged
supernatant fluid.

VIABLE COUNTS OF BACTERIA

A specially devised 4-plate counting technique (6) was used to
count mixtures of the two organisms in 0.1 ml droplets of agar
enriched with 2% lysed horse blood (7) and displayed on a Colworth
Droplette machine (8). Additional droplets were spread on warmed
blood agar plates to provide direct confirmation of the purity and
identify of the bacteria harvested from the wounds.

RESULTS

No technical problems were encountered with the animal model nor
with the preparation, dilution, harvesting or counting of the
organisms.

Studies with pure B.fragilis It proved impossible to induce a
lethal infection in any guinea-pig with B.fragilis, even by
inoculation of its four wounds with an undiluted culture of 9.3 x
10^8 cells per wound. Only at this high concentration was there
any (mild) induration or change in the wound healing. At all lower
inoculum counts there was no macroscopic or histological change to
be observed, although some B.fragilis organisms continued to be
grown from homogenates of the harvested wounds.

Studies with pure E.coli   A fatal E.coli septicaemia was induced regularly with wound inocula containing 10^7 cells or above. When 3×10^6 cells were added to each wound a moderate infection developed within seven days, and for inocula of 3×10^5 cells per wound or below, no inflammation was demonstrable clinically or histologically, at scarifice, a week later, although E.coli could be grown from the healing wound (10^5 cells per wound).

FIGURE 1

Histological Preparation (HE x 10)

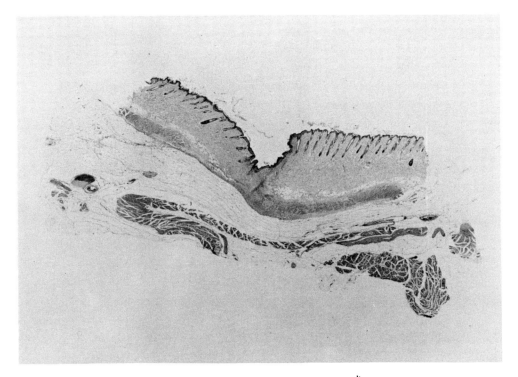

Control wounds and those inoculated with E.coli 9×10^4 cells, or with B.fragilis 9.3×10^4 cells one week earlier all had this appearance.

Studies with mixed inocula of E.coli + B.fragilis Subinfective
doses of each organism were chosen, E.coli 9 x 10^4 cells and
B.fragilis 9.3 x 10^4 cells per wound. Separately, each bacterium
at these concentrations, produced no clinical or histological
effect, and at sacrifice these wounds appeared identical to
uninfected controls (Figure 1). However, when the same total number
of organisms was used in the inocula, half being E.coli (4.5 x 10^4
cells) and half being B.fragilis (4.6 x 10^4 cells),

FIGURE 2

Histological Preparation (HE x 10)

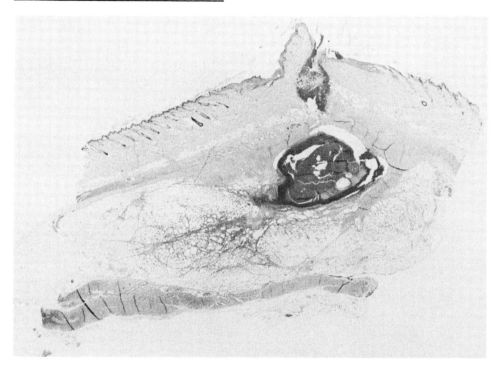

Wound contaminated with mixed E.coli (4.5 x 10^4 cells) plus
B.fragilis (4.6 x 10^4 cells) one week earlier, showing severe
inflammation with pus

at one week the animals were listless, pyrexial (39°C) and unwell, with large swollen wounds filled with frank pus (Figure 2). Wound homogenates showed large and equal numbers of both organisms, E.coli (1.5 x 10^{7} cells) and B.fragilis (2.0 x 10^{7} cells per wound).

The effect of E.coli : B.fragilis ratio on pus formation The concentration of one bacterium in the inoculum was maintained at a constant level (10^{4} cells), whilst that of the second organism varied from 0 to 10^{8} cells (Figure 3). It can be seen that, below a threshold (10^{3} cells of B.fragilis) that bacteroides has no effect on the coliform, and the wound behaves as before (Figure 1), with no infection developing, despite a harvest of 10^{5} cells of E.coli per wound. When the infective mixture contained more than 10^{4} cells of B.fragilis there was synergy with the formation of frank pus containing 10^{7} cells of both organisms.

Similar results were obtained with the reciprocal experiment, except that when E.coli in the inoculum exceeded 10^{5} cells, the animal died of early septicaemia.

Further experiments using differing fixed concentrations of the one bacterium, whilst varying the concentrations of the other, were not done. The possibility of using heat killed bacteria, instead of live organisms, was not investigated.

6

FIGURE 3

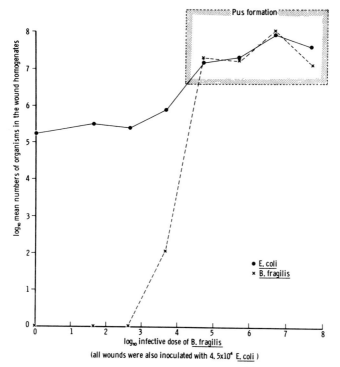

Yields from wound homogenates when challenged with inocula all
containing E.coli (4.5×10^4 cells). The amount of B.fragilis
varied from $0-10^8$ cells.

DISCUSSION

This series of experiments demonstrates synergy between viable
E.coli and B.fragilis in vivo clinically, histologically and
bacteriologically in a quantitative fashion, and has been published
previously (2,9).

Variations in the challenge inocula were minimised by using
thawed ampoules from a single frozen culture batch of each organism,
NCTC reference strain being used. Small volume inocula (0.1 ml)
were used in order to avoid overflowing the wounds which were closed
with standard surgical Michel clips. These appose the wound edges
securely without traversing the tissues themselves, thus avoiding

the problem that stitch material affects the progress of wound infections (10). The suprascapular region of the guinea-pig was chosen as an area with similarities to the human anterior abdominal wall. Each of the four wounds per animal were inoculated with the same concentration of organisms to obviate the problems of disparate wounds affecting each other. The spread-plate feature of the 4-plate counting technique (6) ensured that the organisms seen and counted in the harvested wound homogenate were identical with those E.coli and B.fragilis inoculated one week previously, and were not extraneous contaminants.

Challenge inoculation with this encapsulated NCTC strain of B.fragilis alone, failed to produce any infection, so that in this context it appeared to be "non-pathogenic". The E.coli chosen was pathogenic for guinea-pigs, but only at the higher doses. When a challenge inoculum was used, containing doses of each organism which separately were subinfective, but when they were combined, gave the same total number of organisms i.e. half being E.coli and half B.fragilis, a gross purulent infection resulted allowing the unequivocal demonstration of pathogenic synergy between E.coli and B.fragilis.

The particular E. coli chosen, NCTC9434, was by change, markedly virulent for guinea-pigs, and it may be that the early septicaemic deaths, induced by the larger doses, may have masked an interesting and important area in the synergistic relationship (Dr. H.R. Ingham, personal communication), so further studies using 'weaker' strains might clarify this interaction.

ACKNOWLEDGEMENTS

I am grateful to the Editor of the Journal of Medical Microbiology for permission to reproduce the results of these experiments first published in that journal, and to Dr. B.M. Herbertson, University of Cambridge for review of the slides. This study was supported by grants from the Smith & Nephew Foundation and the East Anglian Regional Health Authority.

8

REFERENCES

1. Kelly MJ & Warren RE. 1978. The value of an operative wound
    swab sent in transport medium in the prediction of later
    clinica wound infection: a controlled clinical and
    bacteriological evaluation. Brit J Surg, 65, 81-89.
2. Kelly MJ. 1978. The quantitative and histological
    demonstration of pathogenic synergy between Escherichia coli
    and Bacteroides fragilis in guinea pig wounds. J Med
    Microbiol, 11, 513-523.
3. Green CJ. 1975. Neuroleptanalgesic drug combinations in the
    anaesthetic management of laboratory small animals. Lab Anims,
    9, 161-178.
4. James JH & Watson ACH. 1975. Use of "Op-Site", a vapour
    permeable dressing, on skin graft donor sites. Brit J Plast
    Surg, 28, 107-110.
5. Sharpe AN & Jackson AK. 1972. Stomaching: a new concept in
    bacteriological sample preparation. Appl Microbiol, 24,
    175-178.
6. Kelly MJ. 1977. Aerobic and anaerobic mixture of human
    pathogens: a rapid 4-plate counting technique. Brit J Exp
    Path, 58, 478-483.
7. Kelly MJ. 1978. Counts on Bacteroides fragilis: a
    modification of the microdroplet technique. J Hyg Camb, 80,
    385-389.
8. Sharpe AN, Dyett EJ, Jackson AK & Kilsby DC. 1972. Technique
    and aparatus for rapid and inexpensive enumeration of
    bacteria. Appl Microbiol, 24, 4-7.
9. Kelly MJ. 1980. Wound infection: a controlled clinical and
    experimental demonstration of synergy between aerobic (E.coli)
    and anaerobic (B.fragilis) bacteria. Annals RCS Eng 62, 52-59.
10. Edlich RF, Rogers W, Kaspar G, Kaufman D, Tsung MS &
    Wangensteen OH. 1969. Studies in the management of the
    contaminated intra-abdominal wound. Amer J Surg, 117, 323-329.

AN ANIMAL MODEL OF PERITONITIS AND THE EFFECT OF ANTI-MICROBIAL
PROPHYLAXIS AND THERAPY

C.E. NORD and G. LAHNBORG

1. INTRODUCTION

   Improved microbiological methods during the last years have
resulted in a widespread appreciation that most intra-abdominal
infections involve both aerobic and anaerobic bacteria. Different
antimicrobial agents have been used for prophylaxis and treatment of
these infections.

   Clinical studies have reported various results for different
types of antimicrobial agents. The approaches in prophylaxis and
treatment vary and it is difficult to evaluate the clinical outcome
of many studies because of host differences, variables in underlying
diseases, the role of surgery and the lack of adequate controls (1).

   The experimental infection in animal models offers an
alternative method for the testing of antimicrobial agents and has
the advantage of allowing evaluation under controlled conditions.

   In order to study the factors involved in peritonitis, a
reproducible experimental model in rats has been developed (2).
This model simulates the intra-abdominal sepsis seen in humans.

   The efficacy of different antimicrobial agents in treatment and
prophylaxis of experimentally induced peritonitis is reported in
this paper.

2. MATERIALS AND METHODS

Animal model

Male Sprague-Dawley rats weighing 180-220 g were used. All animals were housed in individual cages and fed lean ground beef.

The method for producing intraabdominal sepsis described by Lahnborg, Hedstrom and Nord (2) was used. All rats were fasted for 24 h before surgical procedures and then anaesthetized with pentobarbital ("Mebumal", ACO, Stockholm, Sweden) given intraperitoneally at a dosage of 15 mg. The rats were shaved and a midline incision was made. The caecum and terminal part of the ileum were mobilized out of the abdomen. A 2 cm segment of ileum, 5 cm from the ileocaecal junction, was isolated on its vascular pedicle, which was interrupted with a single ligature. The intestine was divided at each end of the segment, and intestinal continuity was reestablished by a one-layer end-to-end anastomosis of the two ends of the ileum using a 6-0 Dexon sutures. The defect in the mesentery was then closed with interrupted 6-0 Dexon sutures. The anastomosis was checked for leakage and passage before the intestine and the devascularized segment of ileum was returned to the abdominal cavity. The abdominal wall was closed in two layers.

Antimicrobial agents

Treatment. Each group consisted of 15 animals. Antimicrobial agents were given by subcutaneous injection, initially, 1 h after surgery and then at 12 h intervals for 10 days. The regimens and amount of agents given per dose were: benzylpenicillin (Astra, Sodertalje, Sweden) 15 mg: piperacillin (Lederle, New York, USA) 40 mg: sulbactam (Pfizer, Sandwich, England) 15 mg: cefoxitin (Merck Sharp and Dohme, Rahway, USA) 20 mg: moxalactam (Lilly,

Indianapolis, USA) 18 mg: thienamycin (Merck Sharpe and Dohme, Rahway, USA) 10 mg: clindamycin (Upjohn, Kalamazoo, USA) 60 mg: metronidazole (May & Baker, Dagenham, England) 3 mg: tinidazole (Pfizer, Sandwich, England) 6 mg: netilmicin (Schering, Bloomfield, USA) 1 mg and fosfomycin (Dumex A/S Cophenagen, Denmark) 60 mg. The control group received 0.9% sterile saline.

Prophylaxis. Each group consisted of 15 animals. All antimicrobials were given subcutaneously immediately before the induction of anaesthesia i.e. half an hour before the operation started. Every animal received only one dosage of antimicrobial or combination of antimicrobials. The amounts of antimicrobials per dose were: doxycycline (Pfizer) 1 mg, cefoxitin 40 mg, metronidazole 3 mg, tinidazole 8 mg plus netilmicin 5 mg, clindamycin 150 mg plus netilmicin 5 mg, cotrimoxazole (Wellcome Foundation, London, England) 60 mg plus tinidazole 8 mg and metronidazole 3 mg plus fosfomycin 60 mg. The control group was given 0.9% sterile saline preoperatively.

Collection and processing of specimens

Specimens were taken with dry cotton-tipped sterile swabs and placed in carbon dioxide-filled glass tubes which were transported to the laboratory as soon as possible. All specimens were streaked on two blood agar plates and ten selective media as described by Heimdahl et al (3). All manipulations of the anaerobic bacteria were carried out in an anaerobic chamber (Forma, Philadelphia, USA) under 10% hydrogen (v/v) in nitrogen. The aerobic agar plates were incubated for 24 h and the anaerobic agar plates for 48 h at 37°C. The plates were then examined and different colony types isolated in pure cultures and identified. The aerobic and anaerobic bacteria were identified by biochemical and serological tests and gas-liquid chromatography (3).

Evaluation of results

Treatment. The following parameters were used for the evaluation of the antimicrobial therapy: mortality rate, time of death and number of abscesses. Autopsies were carried out on all animals.

Prophylaxis. Mortality rate was observed and an autopsy was performed on all animals. The presence of peritoneal fluid, adhesions, distended bowels and abscesses was noted.

3. RESULTS

Treatment

Control group. Within one day, half of the rats were dead and after 4 days 77% of the animals were dead (Fig. 1). All these animals showed typical signs of peritonitis and abscesses when they were autopsied. A polymicrobial flora consisting of Escherichia coli, Proteus mirabilis, Streptococcus faecalis, Bacteroides fragilis, and Clostridium perfringens was recovered from the peritoneal exudate. All rats showed advanced interintestinal adhesions.

Benzylpenicillin. During the first 24 h, 13% of the rats died and for each day up to the fifth day the mortality rate was 18-19% of the total number of animals. All rats that died showed signs of peritonitis. In the peritoneal fluids a mixed microflora with a predominance of E. coli, P. mirabilis, S. faecalis and B. fragilis was found (Fig. 1).

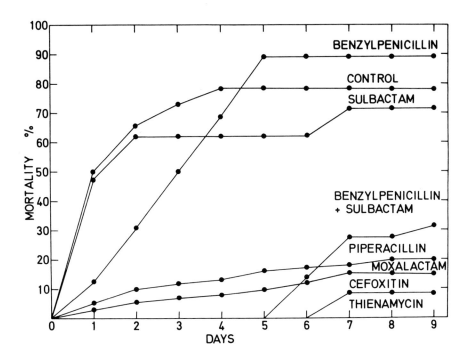

FIGURE 1. Mortality rates in the rats after surgery and either treatment with the indicated antimicrobial agent or no antimicrobial treatment (control). See MATERIALS AND METHODS for doses given.

Sulbactam

The mortality rate (71%) was similar to that found in the control group. E. coli, P. mirabilis, S. faecalis and B. fragilis were recovered from the peritoneal fluids. The rats showed typical signs of peritonitis at autopsy (Fig. 1).

Benzylpenicillin plus sulbactam. The mortality rate was 33%. All animals survived the first five days. In all infected rats an abscess in connection with the anastomosis, was found. E. coli, P. mirabilis and S. faecalis were recovered from the abscesses (Fig. 1).

Piperacillin. All but three rats survived (Fig. 1). At autopsy these animals had abscesses from which E. coli, P. mirabilis, S. faecalis and B. fragilis were recovered.

Cefoxitin. All but one rat survived (Fig. 1). The non-surviving rat died because of ileus, due to a stricture of the anastomosis. All specimens except three showed no growth. S. faecalis in pure culture was isolated from these animals. No sign of previous peritonitis was observed at autopsy.

Moxalactam. Two rats died. From these animals S. faecalis, B. fragilis and C. perfringens were isolated. The surviving animals showed no peritonitis or abscesses at autopsy.

Thienamycin. All animals survived in this group. Thirteen rats had no adhesions or abscesses, two had adhesions, one of which had, in addition, an abscess in the immediate vicinity of the anastomosis. From this abscess E. coli, P. mirabilis, S. faecalis and B. fragilis were cultured. A leakage of the anastomosis was noticed (Fig. 1).

Clindamycin. In this group a marked delay in the mortality rate could be noticed compared to the control group. The overall mortality was 71% (Fig. 2). From the peritoneal fluids only aerobic bacteria (E. coli and P. mirabilis) were isolated. No organisms were isolated from the surviving rats.

Metronidazole. The total mortality rate was 33% (Fig. 2). The signs of peritonitis were less pronounced in this group compared to the control group. Aerobic bacteria (E. coli, P. mirabilis) and S. faecalis were recovered from the infected sites. No organisms were isolated from the surviving rats.

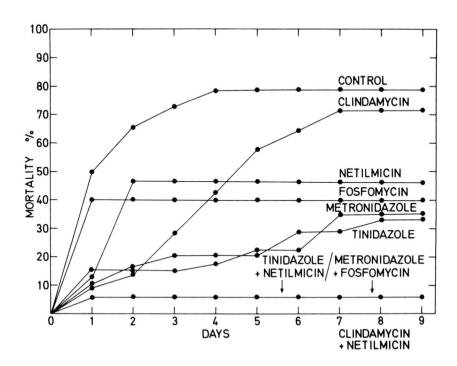

FIGURE 2. Mortality rates in the rats after surgery and either treatment with the indicated antimicrobial agent or no antimicrobial treatment (control). See Materials and Methods for doses given.

Tinidazole. The total mortality rate was 33% (Fig. 2). The signs of peritonitis were similar to those in the metronidazole group. Aerobic bacteria (E. coli, P. mirabilis and S. faecalis) were isolated from the infected sites. No organisms were isolated from the surviving animals.

Fosfomycin. Forty per cent of the rats died within one day (Fig. 2). From the infected sites and the abscesses E. coli, P. mirabilis, S. faecalis, B. fragilis and C. perfringens were cultured.

Netilmicin. Forty-six per cent of the rats died within two days (Fig. 2). E. coli, P. mirabilis, S. faecalis, B. fragilis and C. perfringens were cultured from the infected sites.

Metronidazole plus fosfomycin. All rats except one survived (Fig. 2). At autopsy this animal had an abscess from which E. coli, S. faecalis, and B. fragilis were isolated.

Clindamycin plus netilmicin. All rats survived (Fig. 2). At autopsy one animal had an abscess from which E. coli and S. faecalis were isolated.

Tinidazole plus netilmicin. One animal died (Fig. 2). Abscesses were found in 33% of the rats. E. coli, P. mirabilis, S. faecalis, B. fragilis and C. perfringens were isolated from these abscesses.

Prophylaxis

Control group. The mortality rate is shown in Fig. 3. All animals died within two days and showed, at autopsy, typical signs of acute generalized peritonitis with intraperitoneal. No abscess formation was found. Twelve rats had developed adhesions, primarily around the anastomosis. No rats had distended bowels.

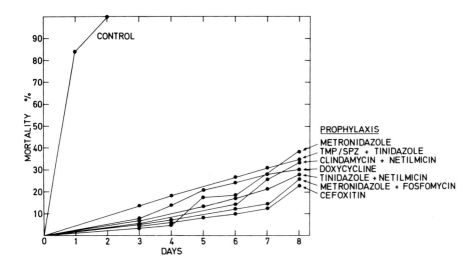

FIGURE 3. Mortality rates in the rats after surgery and either prophylaxis with the indicated antimicrobial agent or no antimicrobial prophylaxis (control). See Materials and Methods for doses given.

Doxycycline. Non-surviving rats showed somewhat less signs of acute peritonitis than the control group (Fig.3). Six rats had intraperitoneal fluid and eight had distended bowels. Twelve rats had adhesions and in nine rats abscesses were observed. No organisms were isolated from the abdominal cavity of one of the surviving rats.

Cefoxitin. Five animals had intraperitoneal fluid and seven had distended bowels (Fig.3). Eight rats had adhesions and in three an abscess was found. The cultures from peritoneal fluid and abscesses showed a polymicrobial flora consisting of E. coli, P.

mirabilis, S. faecalis and B. fragilis. No organisms were isolated from the peritoneal fluid of the surviving rats.

Metronidazole. Six animals had intraperitoneal fluid and distended bowels (Fig.3). Adhesions were found in nine rats and abscesses in two rats. From the infected sites Klebsiella pneumoniae, E. coli, P. mirabilis and S. faecalis were recovered.

Tinidazole plus netilmicin. In this group only three rats had intraperitoneal fluid, though ten had distended bowels (Fig.3). Twelve rats had adhesions and only two had an abscess. From one rat the abdominal content was sterile, whereas the cultures from abscesses and abdominal cavity showed a similar polymicrobial flora comparable to that found in the cefoxitin group.

Metronidazole plus fosfomycin. Similar findings were obtained to the group receiving tinidazole plus netilmicin (Fig.3). Eleven rats had adhesions, two an abscess, nine distended bowels and two had intraperitoneal fluids.

Clindamycin plus netilmicin. Four rats had intraperitoneal fluid, twelve had distended bowels, adhesions were found in twelve and an abscess was found in three (Fig.3). The bacteriology of the peritoneal fluid and abscesses varied markedly: no organisms were isolated from four of the surviving rats, three had S. faecalis only, and E. coli alone was found in one rat which died on the sixth day.

Cotrimoxazole plus tinidazole. Intraperitoneal fluid was not found in this group of fifteen animals. Twelve rats had distended bowels, three had adhesions and abscesses were found in four (Fig.3).

4. DISCUSSION

The present study shows that both aerobic and anaerobic bacteria are involved in intra-abdominal infections. It is, therefore, important to cover for these bacteria with antimicrobial treatment or prophylaxis.

Several of the used antimicrobial combinations proved to be efficient in the treatment of the intra-abdominal sepsis. When benzyl-penicillin was administered alone, no protection against peritonitis was noticed. However, a mixed flora of both aerobes and anaerobes was recovered, which probably means that both bacterial groups can cause peritonitis and death.

Cefoxitin and moxalactam have good *in-vitro* activities against a broad range of aerobic and anaerobic bacteria, including B. fragilis. The present study demonstrated that cefoxitin and moxalactam were effective in treating experimentally-induced intra-abdominal infections.

Piperacillin belongs to the fourth generation of penicillins and has a good *in vitro* activity against a broad range of aerobic and anaerobic bacteria. The present study demonstrated that piperacillin was effective in the treatment of experimentally-induced intra-abdominal infections.

The thienamycin treatment, in the present study, was very favourable. No mortality was observed among the rats.

Sulbactam is a betalactamase inhibitor active against both betalactamases from enterobacteria and B. fragilis. As expected, the inhibitor had no effect on the mortality, or the abscess formation, in the animal experiments. However, when combined with benzylpenicillin a remarkable effect was observed.

Clindamycin has no effect on enterococci and enterobacteria, and therefore aerobic bacteria such as E. coli and P. mirabilis were involved in the development of infection. When clindamycin was combined with netilmicin, cover against both aerobes and anaerobes was obtained and all animals survived.

Metronidazole and tinidazole are only active against anaerobic bacteria in vitro. However, these nitroimidazoles have recently been reported partially to be active against aerobic bacteria in vitro (4,5). This phenomenon can explain the more favourable effect observed on the survival rate with metronidazole and tinidazole therapy than with the clindamycin treatment.

The combination of either metronidazole-fosfomycin or tinidazole-netilmicin resulted in a good response in that only one rat, in each treatment group, died.

When netilmicin was administered alone, a high incidence of death occurred during the two first days. Both aerobes and anaerobes were isolated.

Fosfomycin is a broad-spectrum bactericidal agent which inhibits the cell wall synthesis of both aerobic Gram-positive and Gram-negative bacteria. As expected fosfomycin reduced the mortality rate, but had no effects on abscess formation which is primarily caused by anaerobic bacteria.

Antimicrobial prophylaxis has been generally accepted in surgical practice. Several well-designed and randomized studies have shown that the incidence of postoperative sepsis in patients undergoing colorectal surgery is reduced significantly by antimicrobial prophylaxis (1). Antimicrobial prophylaxis can have an influence on various post-operative changes such as intra-abdominal fluid, adhesions and abscesses. These parameters were studied using the present experimental model.

No significant differences in survival times were noticed for the various antimicrobial agents used. All animals in the control group as well as the non-surviving animals in the other groups, had considerable amounts of intraperitoneal fluid. This finding was not observed in the surviving animals and may be due to the antimicrobial prophylaxis.

The number of adhesions was similar in all groups except in the cefoxitin, the metronidazole and the cotrimoxazole plus tinidazole groups. The incidence of adhesions was relatively high in animals given prophylaxis alone compared with treatment. This may indicate that bacteria play an important part in the development of adhesions. It is possible that antimicrobial agents could also inhibit the development of adhesions.

As expected, the frequency of generally distended bowels was similar in all antimicrobial groups, and is normal postoperative response to surgical trauma.

The incidence of abscesses differed significantly between the doxycycline and the other antimicrobial groups. Aerobic and anaerobic bacteria may not have been susceptible to the dose of doxycycline used.

The present study shows that the selective use of antimicrobial agents is important in the treatment and prophylaxis of intra-abdominal infections. Antimicrobial agents covering both aerobic and anaerobic bacteria should be used.

22

REFERENCES

1. Polk BF. 1981. Antimicrobial prophylaxis to prevent mixed
    bacterial infection. J Antimicrob Chemother. Suppl. D 8:115.

2. Lahnborg G Hedstrom KG, and Nord CE. 1982. Efficacy of
    different antibiotics in the treatment of experimentally-induced
    intra-abdominal sepsis. J Antimicrob Chemother 10:497.

3. Heimdahl A, Kager L, Malmborg AS and Nord CE. 1982. Impact of
    different betalactam antibiotics on the normal human flora and
    colonization of the oral cavity, throat and colon. Infection
    10:120.

4. Ingham HR, Hall CJ, Sisson PR, Tharagonnet D and Selkon JB.
    1980. The activity of metronidazole against facultatively
    anaerobic bacteria. J Antimicrob Chemother. 6:343.

5. Nord CE. 1982. Microbiological properties of tinidazole:
    spectrum, activity and ecological considerations. J Antimicrob
    Chemother, Suppl. A 10:35.

THE PATHOLOGY OF ANIMAL MODELS OF ANTIBIOTIC-ASSOCIATED COLITIS

A. PRICE

INTRODUCTION

In the 1950's when the era of antibiotics began the initial
accounts of antibiotic-associated pseudomembranous colitis (PMC)
suggested that overgrowth by Staphylococcal aureus was the
responsible agent (1). A suitable animal model at that time was
believed to be the chinchilla in whom it was noticed that S. aureus
could be grown from the enteric ulcers that developed after feeding
the animals pellets containing chlortetracycline (2). The vogue for
incriminating S. aureus in human disease waned following the
demonstration that antibiotic-associated PMC occurred with or
without S. aureus present and indeed S. aureus could cause diarrhoea
in the absence of intestinal morphological changes (3).

Renewed interest in antibiotic-associated PMC came in the early
1970's with the flurry of case reports linking lincomycin and
clindamycin with the condition (4, 5). The observation therefore,
that lincomycin also produced a fatal enterocolitis in Syrian golden
hamsters (6) proved to be the foundation for most of the animal
experimental work which then led to the discovery of the aetiology
of PMC (7-10).

HUMAN DISEASE

To appreciate a model requires knowledge of the original, and so
a brief outline of human PMC and the current pathological terminology
is necessary. In man antibiotic-associated PMC refers to a definite
morphological entity characterized by a colo-rectal picture of
varying numbers of adherent mucosal yellow-white plaques (11, 12).
They may be widely spaced or close together, pin-point size or a
coalescing membrane (Fig.1). From observations on surgical
resections and from autopsies, it is known that established disease
involves most of the colon. Segmental involvement can occur and it
is clinically important to realise the rectum can be spared (13).

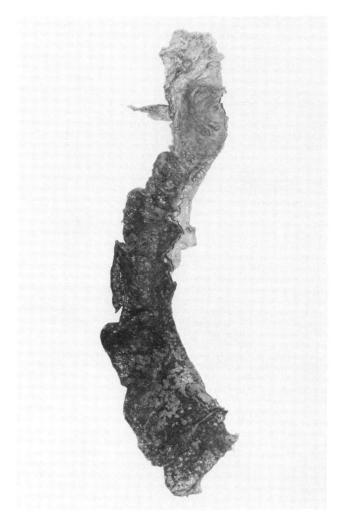

Fig.1   Pseudomembranous colitis in an autopsy specimen. The
         discrete lesions are seen in the upper half of the specimen
         while below the lesions are beginning to coalesce.

Prior to antibiotics small bowel disease was regularly described but
antibiotic-induced disease seems limited to the colon. The
microscopic picture (12) that corresponds with the above is that each
plaque is represented by a well-defined group of disrupted crypts
that have 'disgorged' their contents. The debris, fibrin, mucin and
polymorphs sit as a cap over the dilated lower portions of the crypts
(Fig.2).

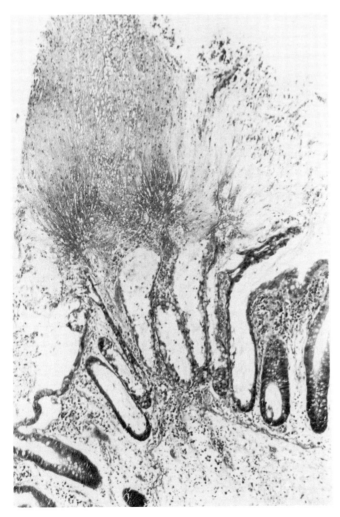

Fig.2   The classical disruptive crypt lesion of pseudomembranous
         colitis. The fibrin, mucus and polymorphonuclear debris on
         the surface forms the yellow plaque (H.E. x 120).

This is the "pseudomembrane". Adjacent mucosa shows important but
only minor focal inflammatory changes and the disease, except in
rare cases of toxic megacolon (14), remains mucosal. In severe
cases the plaques coalesce to form a continuous membrane
representing widespread mucosal necrosis. In very early disease only
tiny focal inflammatory and epithelial changes are present, but
these are relevant to later discussions on the animal model.

For pathologists the stage of a diffuse membrane can no longer be regarded as diagnostic of PMC, as mucosal necrosis is an end stage of many "inflammatory" colonic diseases while the very early focal inflammatory picture, prior to any "disruptive" epithelial changes, is one common to many infective diarrhoea states (15).

CURRENT TERMINOLOGY

The morphological definition of PMC is therefore concise and distinct and within this definition Clostridium difficile and its toxin is involved in up to 97% of cases as the aetiological agent (10). Antibiotic-associated colitis (AAC) and antibiotic-associated diarrhoea (AAD) have a much wider meaning. In AAC, by definition, there must be a histologically proven colitis but it needs not be PMC. Whether a form of AAC exists with a distinct aetiology other than just a "form-truste" of PMC is not clear, although a transient right-sided haemorrhagic colitis due to penicillin derivatives has been described (16). AAD (with no proven mucosal histological abnormality) encompasses a much wider clinical spectrum, and C. difficile is involved in only some 6% of cases (10). If one is limited by those morphological considerations then, while there are many animal models for AAC, there are but few, if any, of PMC. Despite disappointment for pathologists much has been learnt from animal work about the microbiology and epidemiology of the disease.

THE HAMSTER MODEL (experimental observations)

After the observation by Larson et al. (7) that a toxin was present in the stool of patients with antibiotic-associated PMC the subsequent unravelling of the story evolved through affected patients in parallel with the experimental situation in the Syrian hamster. The base line observation being that the majority of hamsters kept under normal cage conditions develop a fatal enterocolitis 2-5 days after an oral or peritoneal challenge with clindamycin or lincomycin (6). The caecal contents of hamsters dying with clindamycin - or lincomycin - induced enterocolitis contain a toxin identical to that in the stools of patients with PMC (17). This was next shown to be derived from C. difficile (9) but, at first, workers were mislead as the toxin cross reacts with C. sordellii antitoxin (18).

C. difficile is only rarely found in healthy humans and this holds true for the hamster model (19). The caecal contents, or cell free filtrates, from diseased animals will also reproduce the enterocolitis if inoculated into healthy animals either via an orogastric tube or directly into the caecum (20). Stool suspensions or cell free filtrates from humans with PMC will produce an identical picture if inoculated into hamsters (21). Broth cultures of caecal isolates of C. difficile from hamsters dying with AAC will also produce a caecitis in hamsters (20). However, if such cultures are washed free of toxin then administered by orogastric tube, disease will only occur if the hamster has been pretreated with antibiotics (21). This situation is akin to the human where in the majority of cases the bowel must first be made susceptible to colonization by a course of antibiotics.

Other microbiological data has been built up via protection experiments. For example, administration of C. sordellii antitoxin to hamsters will protect against clindamycin-induced disease (22). Incubation of the caecal contents of a diseased animal with C. sordellii antitoxin prevents disease when these contents are inoculated into a healthy animal (20).

Similar to human PMC many antibiotics will induce disease in the hamster (9) and again bearing similarity to the human situation vancomycin has a protective role (23). However the animals do show an increased state of susceptibility once the vancomycin is withdrawn with disease developing subsequently at intermittent intervals over a period of one to two weeks (24). If the experiment is carried out under sterile conditions disease does not occur. In a series of experiments using sterile cages and housing hamsters in various "clean or dirty" areas of a hospital and animal house Larson et al. (19) showed that the animals could survive antibiotic challenge if kept free of exposure to C. difficile, and if exposed would only succumb if pre-treated with antibiotics.

The sum of this experimental data has been to show that C. difficile and its toxins are the cause of antibiotic-associated caecitis in the hamster and that it appears to be an infectious disease. The bowel must first be made susceptible to colonization.

The microbiology and epidemiology of human AAC and/or PMC is virtually identical (19, 25).

PATHOLOGY OF THE HAMSTER MODEL

Turning to the comparative morphology of human versus hamster disease differences emerge (26, 27). Unlike human PMC the experimental disease only affects the caecum and the classical yellow "paint-blob" lesions are not seen. One of two patterns predominate. Macroscopically the caecum is either grossly dilated and haemorrhagic or remains close to normal size but the wall has a thickened velvety texture with some haemorrhagic spots (Fig.3).

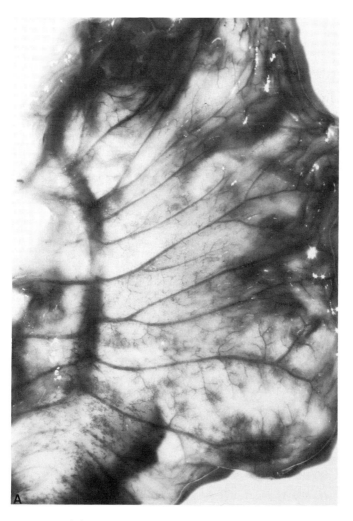

Fig.3   (a) Left: Part of a normal hamster caecum to demonstrate the translucency of the wall.

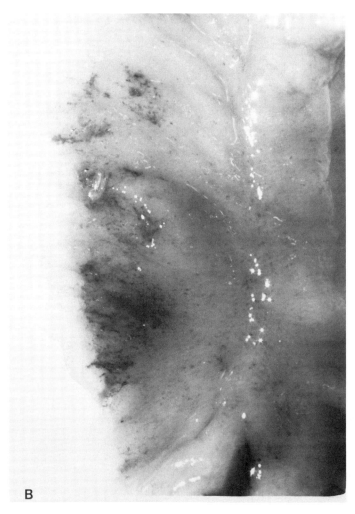

Fig.3 (b) Right The thickened caecal wall from a hamster with antibiotic-induced colitis.

On microscopy (26, 27) animals with caecal dilatation show gross mucosal haemorrhage, the caecal glands surviving in the background of free blood (Fig. 4).

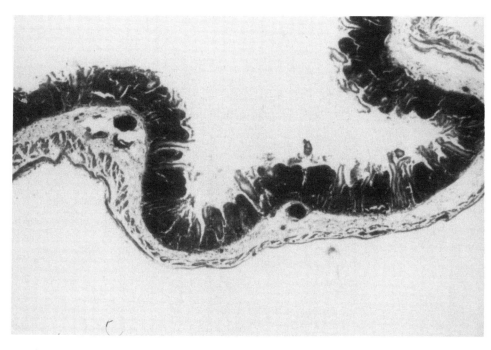

Fig.4   The haemorrhagic pattern of pathology in the caecum of a hamster with clindamycin-induced caecitis (H.E. x 50).

Those with a thickened caecum show a marked increase in mucosal depth due to crypt elongation with surface epithelial proliferation and degenerative changes. There is accompanying focal inflammation mainly limited to the mucosa (Fig.5).

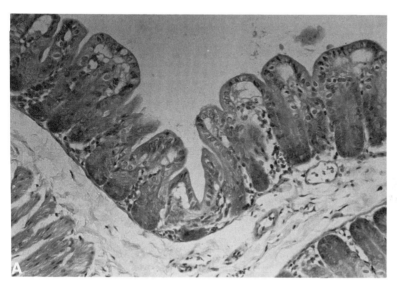

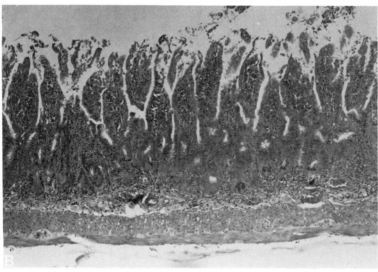

Fig.5   (a) Upper -   Normal hamster caecal mucosa for comparison with (b).

            (b) Lower -   The thickened mucosa (4b, right) showing crypt elongation and some inflammation from a hamster dying with clindamycin-induced caecitis (H.E. x 240).

Ulceration is a variable finding and the ulcer slough should not be equated with a pseudomembrane. Sometimes the changes extend into the terminal ileum and, at this site, the picture can become confused with "wet-tail" or proliferative ileitis (28), a naturally occurring entity in hamster colonies but not associated with the isolation of clostridial organisms. Gram staining in antibiotic-induced disease shows a mixed collection of positive and negative organisms all limited to the mucosal surface. Figures 2, 4 and 5 show that morphologically the comparative microscopy has only limited similarities. Furthermore the hamster lesions are invariably caecal. These differences may be for reasons unique to hamster or human micro-anatomy or because of our inadequate knowledge about the pathogenesis of the lesions. Either way there is still a need to find an animal in which a more exact replica of human colonic disease is produced.

It is interesting to note that in human AAC (with no pseudomembranes) the minor mucosal abnormalities present are very similar to changes present in sub-clinical disease in the hamster (15). Animals challenged with clindamycin and then non-pathogenic C. difficile are protected from subsequent challenge by pathogenic strains as shown by Borriello and Barclay (this volume). The caecal mucosa in such animals is seen in Fig.6 and resembles that observed in toxin-positive patients with AAC and, indeed, in patients with any mild attack of bacterial colitis (29). The variations in pathological picture in the hamster could be equivalent to the spectrum of antibiotic-associated disease seen in the human which was discussed earlier. The appreciation that strains of C. difficile differ in their pathogenecity must also influence the final pathology.

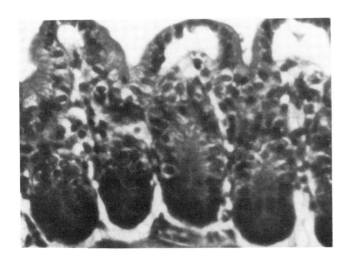

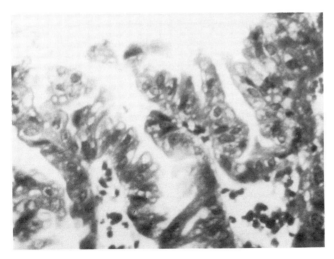

Fig.6   The normal caecal mucosa with its smooth outline is seen
        above in contrast to the tufted and vacuolated epithelium
        below from a hamster colonized by non-pathogenic
        C.difficile after a clindamycin challenge (H.E. x 320).

C.Difficile toxins

It is now known that some of the variation between strains of
C. difficile could be related to the presence of two toxins (30).
These are toxin A, an 'enterotoxin' and toxin B, a cytotoxin. There
are no pathological observations in humans on the separate effects
of the toxins to date and there is still considerable technical
difficulty in obtaining pure preparations. It would be satisfactory
if the two patterns of caecal pathology in hamsters described above
(27) could be related to each of the toxins. This seems unlikely
since Libby et al. (31) demonstrated some differences in
pathological response between the cytotoxin and enterotoxin, they
were quantitative and not clear cut. It is toxin A that produces a
positive response in the rabbit ileal loop and is presumably
responsible for water influx with consequences on the pathogenesis
of diarrhoea. Either toxin is lethal to the hamster and only
protection against both prevents the fatal outcome of a clindamycin
challenge. Future work on the role of each toxin promises much
towards understanding the pathogenesis of antibiotic C. difficile
induced colitis.

OTHER ANIMAL MODELS

Because of the morphological limitations of the hamster model
and the difficulty in obtaining monocontaminated animals, other
models have been sought. An antibiotic-induced enterocolitis has
been produced in guinea-pigs (32), rabbits (33), hares (34), rats
(35) and mice (36) with varying degrees of success. In some
experiments, germ-free species have been used.

A haemorrhagic caecitis in response to penicillin and from which
C. difficile has been isolated is described by Lowe et al. (32). In
rabbits an iota toxin thought to be produced by C. perfringens type
E was detected in response to antibiotics by La Mont et al. (33) but
Dabard and colleagues (34) claimed that C. difficile will not
colonize young rabbits. It is possible that another clostridium,
C. spiroforme has a role in enteritis of the rabbit (37) indeed the
toxin of C. spiroforme cross reacts with C. perfringens type E
antitoxin.

<u>Clostridium difficile</u> was associated with diarrhoea in young conventional and gnotobiotic hares (34). It also produces disease in young conventional and gnotobiotic hares (34). It also produces disease in monoassociated rats (35). The latter may prove a useful model to the pathologist, as there is widespread colonic involvement although the ulceration is not quite typical of human PMC. Prior to the discovery of the role of <u>C. difficile</u> in PMC it had been shown that germ free rats develop antibodies to colonic mucosa if contaminated with the organism (38). In gnotobiotic mice the response to colonization by <u>C. difficile</u> seems variable, with some reports of a mild chronic diarrhoea (36) but other reports of no effect (34).

CONCLUSIONS

In summary, the hamster has provided a wealth of bacteriological and epidemiological data as a model of AAC but there are morphological limitations when compared to PMC. At the present time no other animal model has been shown to be more useful. Now that the basic data on the role of <u>C. difficile</u> has been established a good model is required on which there can be controlled manipulation of the intestinal environment. One of the main questions still outstanding is to discover the exact mechanism that allows the normal colon to be colonized by <u>C. difficile</u>.

REFERENCES

1. Terplan K, Paine JR, Sheffer J, Egan R, Lansky. (1953). Fulminating gastroenterocolitis caused by <u>staphylococci</u>; its apparent connection with antibiotic medication. Gastroenterology <u>24</u>: 476-509.

2. Wood JS, Bennett IL, Yardley JH. (1956). Staphylococcal enterocolitis in chinchillas. Bull. John Hopkins Hosp. <u>98</u>, 454-463.

3. Dearing WH, Baggenotoss AH, Weed LA. (1960). Studies on the relationship of <u>Staphylococcus aureus</u> to pseudomembranous enteritis and post-antibiotic enteritis. Gastroenterology <u>38</u>, 441-451.

4. Cohen LE, McNeill CJ, Wells RF. (1973). Clindamycin-associated colitis. J.Am.Med.Ass. <u>223</u>, 1379-1380.

5. Scott AJ, Nicholson GI, Kerr AR. (1973). Lincomycin as a cause of pseudomembranous colitis. Lancet 2, 1232-1234.

6. Small JD. (1968). Fatal enterocolitis in hamsters given lincomycin hydrochloride. Lab. Animal Care 18, 411-420.

7. Larson HE, Parry JV, Price AB, Davies DR, Dolby J, Tyrell DAJ. (1977). Undescribed toxin in pseudomembranous colitis. Lancet i, 1063-1066.

8. Bartlett JG, Chang TW, Gurwith M, Gorbach SL, Onderdonk AB. (1978). Antibiotic-associated pseudomembranous colitis due to toxin-producing clostridia. New Eng.J.Med. 298, 531-534.

9. Bartlett JG, Chang TW, Moon N, Onderdonk AB. (1978). Antibiotic-induced lethal enterocolitis in hamsters: studies with eleven agents and evidence to support the pathogenic role of toxin producing clostridia. Am.J.Vet.Res. 39, 1525-1530.

10. Bartlett JG, Moon N, Chang TW, Taylor N, Onderdonk A.B. (1978). Role of Clostridium difficile in antibiotic-associated pseudomembranous colitis. Gastroenterology 75, 778-782.

11. Goulston SJM, McGovern VJ. (1965). Pseudomembranous colitis, Gut 6, 207-212.

12. Price AB, Davies DR. (1977). Pseudomembranous colitis. J.Clin.Pathol. 30, 1-12.

13. Tedesco FJ, Corless JK, Brownstein RE. (1982). Rectal sparing in antibiotic-associated pseudomembranous colitis: a prospective study. Gastroenterology 83, 1259-1260.

14. Cone JB, Wetzel W. (1982). Toxin megacolon secondary to pseudomembranous colitis. Dis.Col.Rect. 25, 478-482.

15. Price AB, Day DW. (1982). Pseudomembranous and infective colitis. In Recent Advances in Histopathology II. ed. Anthony, P.P., MacSween, R.N.M., Edinburgh Churchill Livingstone. Pp.99-117.

16. Gould PC, Khawaza FI, Rosenthal WS. (1982). Antibiotic-associated haemorrhagic colitis. Am.J.Gastroenterology 77, 491-493.

17. Bartlett JG, Onderdonk AB, Cisneros RL, Kapser DL. (1977). Clindamycin-associated colitis due to toxin producing species of Clostridium in hamsters. J.Infect.Dis. 136, 701-705.

18. Rifkin GD, Fekety FR, Silva J.Jr. (1977). Antibiotic-induced colitis, implication of a toxin neutralised by Clostridium sordellii antitoxin. Lancet ii, 1103-1106.

19. Larson HE, Price AB, Borriello SP. (1980). Epidemiology of experimental enterocolitis due to Clostridium difficile. The J.Infect.Dis. 142, 408-413.

20. Rifkin GD, Silva J, Fekety R. (1978). Gastrointestinal and systemic toxicity of fecal extracts from hamsters with clindamycin-induced colitis. Gastroenterology 74, 52-57.

21. Larson HE, Price AB, Honour P, Borriello SP. (1978). Clostridium difficile and the aetiology of pseudomembranous colitis. Lancet i, 1063-1066.

22. Allo M, Silva J.Jr, Fekety R, Rifkin G, Waskin H. (1979). Prevention of clindamycin-induced colitis in hamsters by Clostridium sordellii antitoxin. Gastroenterology 76, 351-355.

23. Bartlett JG, Onderdonk AB, Cisneros RL, (1977[a]). Clindamycin-associated colitis in hamsters: protection with vancomycin. Gastroenterology 73, 772-776.

24. Toshniwal R, Silva J.Jr, Fekety R, Kyung-Hee K. (1981). Studies on the epidemiology of colitis due to Clostridium difficile in hamsters. The J.Infect.Dis. 143, 51-54.

25. Greenfield C, Burroughs A, Szawathowski M, Bass N, Noone P, Pounder R. (1981). Is pseudomembranous colitis infectious? Lancet i, 371-372.

26. Humphrey CD, Lushbaugh WB, Condon CW, Pittman JC, Pittman FE. (1979). Light and electron microscopic studies of antibiotic-associated colitis in the hamster. Gut 20, 6-15.

27. Price AB, Larson HE, Crow J. (1979b). Morphology of experimental antibiotic-associated enterocolitis in the hamster: a model for human pseudomembranous colitis and antibiotic-associated colitis. Gut 20, 467-475.

28. Jacoby RO. (1978). Transmissable ileal hyperplasia of hamsters. Amer.J.Pathol. 91, 433-450.

29. Price AB, Jewkes J, Sanderson PJ. (1979a). Acute diarrhoea: Campylobacter colitis and the role of rectal biopsy. J.Clin.Pathol. 32, 990-997.

30. Taylor NS, Thorne GM, Bartlett JG. (1981). Comparison of two toxins produced by Clostridium difficile. Infect.Imm. 34, 1036-1043.

31. Libby JM, Jortner BS, Wilkins TD. (1982). Effects of two toxins of Clostridium difficile in antibiotic-associated cecitis in hamsters. Infect.Imm. 36, 822-829.

32. Lowe BR, Fox JG, Bartlett JG. (1980). Clostridium difficile-associated cecitis in guinea pigs exposed to penicillin. Am.J.Vet. 41, 1277-1279.

33. La Mont JT, Sonnenbluck EB, Rothman S. (1979). Role of clostridial toxin in the pathogenesis of clindamycin colitis in rabbits. Gastroenterology 76, 356-361.

34. Dabard J, Dubos F, Martinet L, Duchizeau R. (1979). Experimental reproduction of neonatal diarrhoea in young gnotobiotic hares simultaneously associated with Clostridium difficile and other Clostridium strains. Infect.Imm. 24, 7-11.

35. Czuprynski CJ, Johnson WJ, Balish E, Wilkin T. (1983). Pseudomembranous colitis in Clostridium difficile-monoassociated rats. Infect.Imm. 39, 1368-1376.

36. Onderdonk AB, Cisneros RL, Bartlett JG. (1980). Clostridium difficile in Gnotobiotic Mice. Infect.Imm. 28, 277-282.

37. Boriello SP, Carman RJ. (1983). Association of iota-like toxin and Clostridium spiroforme with both spontaneous and antibiotic-associated diarrhoea and colitis in rabbits. J.Clin.Microbiol. 17, 414-418.

38. Hammarstrom SP, Perlmann BE, Gustaffson BE, Lagercranty R. (1969). Autoantibodies to colon in germfree rats monocontaminated with Clostridium difficile. J.Exp.Med. 129, 747-756.

BACTEROIDES FRAGILIS, PROPIONIBACTERIUM ACNES AND PEPTOSTREPTOCOCCUS
ANAEROBIUS IN EXPERIMENTAL OTITIS MEDIA IN GUINEA-PIGS.

MAGNUS THORE, LARS G. BURMAN, STIG E. HOLM.

SUMMARY

A guinea-pig model for induction of otitis-media by anaerobic
bacteria is described. Bacteroides fragilis (4-8x10^7 colony forming
units) injected via the tympanic membrane was capable of inducing
intense inflammation with persisting sequelae and survived for at
least 21 days in the middle ear cavity of the animals.
Propionibacterium acnes also induced otitis media although not as
intense and protracted as the B.fragilis infection. The middle ear
response to experimentally inoculated Peptostreptococcus anaerobius
was weak and transitory.

INTRODUCTION

In recent years non-spore-forming anaerobic bacteria have become
increasingly recognized as significant pathogens in upper respiratory
tract infections. For example, the presence of anaerobic bacteria in
addition to aerobic bacteria is well documented in samples of effusion
from middle ears with chronic discharge (1, 2). Bacteroides species
(including B.fragilis) and peptococci dominated the anaerobic
component but Propionibacterium acnes was also found. Furthermore,
anaerobic bacteria in pure culture have recently been isolated from
9-13% of samples of middle ear effusion from children with acute,
purulent otitis media (3). The anaerobic species found in middle ear
and in paranasal sinus effusions (4, 5) are also isolated from the
therapeutically difficult brain abscesses that occasionally complicate
such infections (6). These findings further emphasize the virulence
of anaerobic bacteria in upper respiratory tract infections.

Nitroimidazole therapy against the anaerobes isolated has been tried in patients with middle ear disease (7) or with other upper respiratory tract infections (8). However, the results concerning acute middle ear infections were disappointing (7).

With regard to the risk of serious complications in otitis and sinusitis such as brain abscess and the uncertainty regarding the proper treatment of the anaerobic focal infection, it is important to define an animal model in which monoinfections in the middle ear with different species of anaerobic bacteria can be induced and studied. This paper describes a guinea-pig model for anaerobic otitis media and used to evaluate the capacity of B.fragilis, P.acnes and Peptostreptococcus anaerobius to cause inflammation and survive in the middle ear.

MATERIALS AND METHODS

Preparation of challenge organisms

A bacterial suspension was prepared using bacteria growing under anaerobic conditions (GasPak system, BBL, Cockeysville, Md) on the surface of blood agar plates (OXOID, London) that had been inoculated 48 hours earlier. The strains used were B. fragilis NCTC 9343, Propionibacterium acnes NCTC 737 and Peptostreptococcus anaerobius ATCC 27337. Virulence of B.fragilis was maintained by using bacteria from previously infected guinea-pigs in the succeeding experiment. Immediately before an experiment the bacteria were harvested, washed once, and resuspended in buffer. The buffer contained 130 mM KCl, 2 mM $MgSO_4$ and 50 mM HEPES (Sigma Chemical Co., St.Louis) in deionized water and was adjusted to pH 7.5 with KOH. The turbidity of the bacterial suspensions was adjusted to the desired challenge dose using a Vitatron spectrophotometer (Hugo Tillqvist AB, Stockholm). The suspensions were then aspirated into the 1 ml syringes used for inoculation.

Induction of otitis media in guinea-pigs

Healthy albino guinea-pigs (Nybergs Gard, Marsta, Sweden, 6-24 weeks old, weight 250-450 g) were used. The animals were kept in individual ventilated cages.

Before an experiment the animals were anaesthetized by an ip injection of 30 mg of pentobarbital/kg bodyweight, and both ears were examined to exclude infections. The right external ear, including the external ear canal, was disinfected using 10% hydrogen peroxide for 30 sec followed by 3% iodine in 70% ethanol for 30 sec. The iodine was inactivated by sterile 10% sodium thiosulphate and a final wash with sterile water was performed. Culture negative swabs from the ears were obtained from all animals after this disinfection procedure.

The bacterial suspension (0.1-0.2 ml) was injected through the tympanic membrane into the right middle ear, leaving the left ear as an uninoculated control. In order to reduce later contamination the external ear canal was sealed with a plug consisting of paraffin and petroleum jelly.

It has been noted previously that injection of sterile HEPES buffer into the middle ear of guinea-pigs often causes inflammation (probably because of invasion of bacteria from the nasopharynx). In all challenge experiments a daily ip injection of 4.5 mg of gentamicin (Schering Corp. Kenilworth, N.J.) in 1 ml of sterile water was used as prophylaxis against aerobic superinfection (9).

Sacrifice of guinea-pigs and bacteriological sampling of ears

At various intervals after bacterial challenge, the animals were killed using a lethal dose of pentobarbital. The external ears were removed and the temporal bones were surgically separated from the skull. The middle ears were entered through an infero-posterior hole that was made using a pair of sterile bone tongs. After gross examination of the middle ears, any effusion present was aspirated and immediately diluted into 5 ml of phosphate-buffered saline (PBS, 12.6 mM KH_2PO_4, 54.0 mM Na_2HPO_4, 85 mM NaCl, pH 7.4). The middle ears were then washed with 0.1-0.2 ml of PBS using the same syringe, and the wash fluid was added to the specimen. After appropriate dilutions the samples were spread over blood agar plates (OXOID) and immediately incubated anaerobically (GasPak) and aerobically for 48 hours at $37°C$. The colonies obtained were counted and identified by morphology and according to Holdeman and

co-workers (10). Aerobic bacteria were identified according to
standard techniques. The control (left) middle ears never showed
signs of infection.

Microscopic examination of ears

Representative ears were fixed in 10% neutral formaldehyde and
decalcified in New Decalk^R (Histo-Lab. Bethlehem Trading,
Gothenburg) for 4-5 hrs. After dehydration the material was
embedded in paraffin and sectioned. The thin sections were stained
with hematoxylin and eosin before light microscopy.

RESULTS

Inoculation of low doses of bacteria

In preliminary experiments 10^5 colony forming units (cfu) were
used as challenge dose. However, the counts of P.acnes (NCTC 737)
recovered on day 5 after challenge were low and minimal, or no
otitis reaction was noted. The same dose of B.fragilis (NCTC 9343)
or Peptostreptococcus anaerobius (ATCC 27337) did not induce otitis
media and no bacteria were recovered on day 5. The challenge dose
was therefore increased to $4-8 \times 10^7$ cfu/ear for all bacterial
species in the experiments reported below.

Inoculation of B.fragilis (NCTC 9343)

Forty-four animals were challenged with B.fragilis and studied
after 3, 5, 10, 12, 18, 21 or 35 days. On day 3, 5, 10 and 12
B.fragilis was isolated as a single species from 20 of 28 ears
studied. Only one of the eight ears not yielding B.fragilis was
invaded by another microorganism (enterococci). B.fragilis was
still cultivable at later stages. On day 18 and 21 pure cultures of
B.fragilis were obtained from 7 of 12 ears sampled. In addition,
B.fragilis together with staphylococci and enteric bacilli were
cultured from the middle ear of another animal. B.fragilis was not
isolated on day 35, after challenge, whereas from one of the four
ears, staphylococci and alpha-hemolytic streptococci were recovered.

The elimination of B.fragilis from the middle ear was slow, although an individual variability was noted (Fig.1). Some animals seemed to eliminate B.fragilis at an early stage whereas, in the majority of ears, the counts were relatively stable ($3.5 \times 10^4 - 10^6$ cfu/ear) during the first 12 days followed by gradual decline. In 4 of 12 ears the counts remained stable even during the third week after challenge.

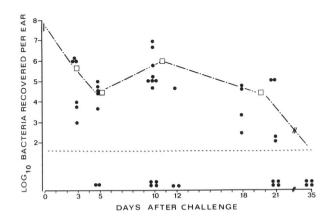

Fig. 1. Recovery of Bacteroides fragilis (NCTC 9343) from the right middle ears of 44 guinea-pigs on various days after inoculation. Closed circles represent total counts for individual ears, open squares denote arithmetic mean values. On day 0, the bacteria ($4-8 \times 10^7$ colony forming units, cfu) suspended in buffer (see Materials and Methods) were injected through the tympanic membrane into the right middle ear cavity. Bacterial counts less than 50 cfu per ear were not detected under the assay conditions employed, and such ears were recorded as culture negative (below dashed line).

The inflammatory response to B.fragilis challenge was pronounced, at the bacterial dose applied. On day 3, purulent effusion was noted in 5 of 6 ears studied. On day 5, 4 of 7 ears studied contained small amounts of purulent effusion and 3 ears were inflamed but dry. On day 10 and 12, 10 of 15 ears studied contained varying amounts of purulent effusion. The inflammatory reaction was usually less pronounced on day 18 and 21. On day 35 small amounts of effusion were noted in one ear and B.fragilis was not recovered in any of the 4 ears cultured.

44

About one third of the inoculated ears were also studied
histologically. During the early phase of infection the histological
picture was dominated by subepithelial oedema and infiltration by
inflammatory cells, mainly polymorphonuclear leukocytes. Profuse new
bone formation with extensive growth of periosteum was evident in
culture-positive ears on day 10-12 (Fig. 2) and was still present on
day 35 (Fig. 3). The new bone formation was further recognized as an
increased difficulty in surgical penetration into the cavity.

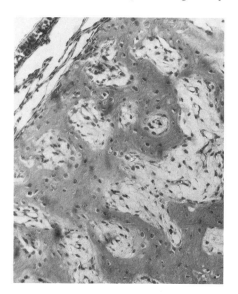 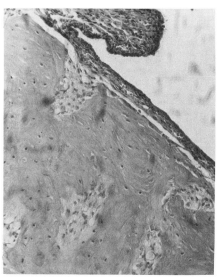

Fig. 2. Light micrograph of the
sectioned middle ear of a guinea-
pig challenged with B.fragilis
(NCTC 9343) 12 days earlier.
Note the profuse new bone
formation (dark areas) with
extensive growth of periosteum as
granulation tissue in the bone.
Hematoxylin and eosin x 200.

Fig. 3. Light micrograph of the
sectioned middle ear of a guinea-
pig challenged with B.fragilis
(NCTC 9343) 35 days earlier.
Newly formed bone with islands
of granulation tissue is still
visible. The subepithelium is
thickened and occasionally
forming polyps (upper margin).
Hematoxylin and eosin x 200.

In 11 of 44 ears included in this B.fragilis series, the tympanic
membrane was perforated at the time of sacrifice. No signs of
labyrinthitis were noted and none of the animals showed behavioural
abnormalities suggesting other complications during the observation
period.

Inoculation of P.acnes (NCTC 737) and Peptostreptococcus anaerobius (ATCC 27337)

Twenty-eight animals were challenged with P.acnes and studied
after 3, 5, 10, 12 or 35 days. On day 3, 5 and 10 P.acnes was
isolated as single species from 15 of 21 ears studied. P.acnes was
isolated from 3 additional ears, one of which also contained aerobic
diphtheroid rods. In the two others with beta-hemolytic
streptococci were isolated. The counts of P.acnes recovered from
the middle ears declined from 10^5 on day 3 to 2×10^2 cfu on day
10 (Fig. 4). On day 12 P.acnes was not recovered, but secondary
invasion had occurred in 2 of 3 ears (by staphylococci and
beta-hemolytic streptococci, respectively). On day 35 no bacteria
were recovered from the 4 ears studied.

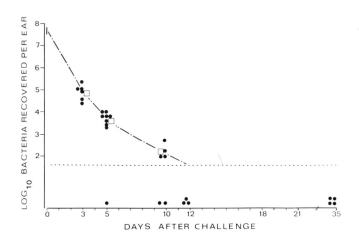

Fig. 4. Recovery of P.acnes (NCTC 737) from the right middle ears
of 28 guinea-pigs on various days after inoculation. For further
explanation, see Fig. 1.

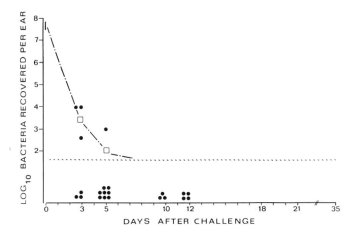

Fig. 5. Recovery of Peptostreptococcus anaerobius (ATCC 27337) from the right middle ears of 22 guinea-pigs on various days after inoculation. For further explanation, see Fig. 1.

Moderate amounts of serous or purulent effusion was noted on day 3 and 5 in 8 of 15 ears, whereas the remaining ears showed negligible signs of otitis media. The histological picture during the initial phase of P.acnes otitis was dominated by subepithelial oedema with inflammatory cells. On day 10 and 12 the otitis reaction was less pronounced, although slight amounts of effusion were noted in 2 ears that had not been secondarily invaded. On day 35 no signs of sequelae were noted except in one ear showing slight mucoperiostial thickening with new bone formation. Of the 28 ears included in this P.acnes series, four tympanic membranes were perforated at the time of sacrifice. None of the animals showed behavioural abnormalities and no histological signs of labyrinthitis were noted.

Among the 22 animals challenged with P.anaerobius and studied after 3, 5, 10 or 12 days, rapid elimination of the challenge organism occurred (Fig. 5). On day 3 and 5 P.anaerobius was isolated as single organism from only 3 of the 15 ears studied. The organism was found together with aerobic diphtheroid rods in another ear on day 3. The challenge organism was never recovered on day 10 or 12 (Fig. 5). Inoculation of P.anaerobius was associated with, at best, a weak inflammatory response and already, on day 5, little or no sign of inflammation was noted in ears that had not been exposed to secondary invaders. No behavioural abnormalities or histological signs of labyrinthitis were noted in the P.anaerobius series.

DISCUSSION

The present data demonstrate that B.fragilis as well as P.acnes can survive and induce an inflammatory reaction when introduced into the middle ear of the guinea-pig. Peptostreptococcus anaerobius on the other hand failed to induce otitis media in this model. The virulence of P.acnes is in agreement without earlier study (9) where higher doses of this organism were found to induce an otitis reaction very similar to that seen after challenge with Streptococcus pneumoniae (type 23F), a classic middle ear pathogen in humans. The shortcoming of peptostreptococci in this model is also in agreement with our previous experiments where Peptostreptococcus micros failed to induce otitis media in guinea-pigs. Also Bacteroides asaccharolyticus was unable to induce otitis in guinea-pigs (9). In contrast, B.fragilis caused a typical otitis media, clinically, bacteriologically, as well as histologically.

Fulghum et al. (11) used the Mongolian gerbil for experimental induction of otitis media. These authors used a clinical isolate of P.acnes and challenge doses similar to those used to induce otitis media in the present study. They reported both otoscopic and histopathological evidence of P.acnes infection similar to our results in guinea-pigs. However, in contrast to the guinea-pigs the gerbils also showed behavioural symptoms.

Using a challenge dose of $4-8 \times 10^7$ cfu, P.acnes otitis was not as intense and persistent as the B.fragilis otitis. Elimination of P.acnes was completed within 12 days, whereas B.fragilis was still cultivable 21 days after challenge. The histological examination revealed an intense infection with persisting sequelae, i.e. new bone formation, even 35 days after B.fragilis challenge. B.fragilis did, however, not induce labyrinthitis in our model. This complication reportedly occurs in B.fragilis otitis in humans (7) and is frequently seen in experimental pneumococcal otitis media in guinea-pigs (12). Thus, the response to various middle ear pathogens seems to depend on the bacterial species or strain studied and also differs between animal species.

The earlier experimental problem, a frequent development of
otitis media following injection of only sterile buffer into the
middle ear of the guinea-pig, was overcome by a daily ip injection
of gentamicin (9). This complication would not seem to occur in
experimental otitis in chinchillas (13, 14). Although we have not
been fully successful in eliminating secondary invaders so far the
present incidence of superinfection (less than 10%) does not
invalidate the interpretation of the results.

In order to further characterize our otitis model we are
currently investigating the development of serum antibodies against
the present challenge organisms. Preliminary results obtained with
an indirect immunofluorescence test suggest that P.acnes and
Ps.anaerobius do not cause development of serum antibodies belonging
to any of the main immunoglobulin (IgG, IgM or IgA). In contrast,
B.fragilis otitis seems to evoke a strong and specific IgG and IgM
response.

In conclusion, we have shown that classical otitis media can be
experimentally induced in guinea-pigs by anaerobic bacteria, notably
B.fragilis. This animal model might be useful in studies of
antimicrobial therapy in anaerobic otitis media.

ACKNOWLEDGMENTS

We thank Wigert Sjoberg, Stig Granstrom and Siw Domeij for
technical assistance. Grants were obtained from the Medical
Faculty, University of Umea and from the Mangberg and the Arner
foundations.

REFERENCES

1. Jokipii RMM, Karma P, Ojala K and Jokipii L. 1977. Anaerobic
   bacteria in chronic otitis media. Arch. Otolaryng. 103, 278-280.

2. Sugita R, Kawamura S, Ichikawa G, Gato S and Fujimaki Y. 1981.
   Studies on anaerobic bacteria in chronic otitis media.
   Laryngoscope 91, 816-821.

3. Brook I. 1979. Otitis media in children: a prospective study
   of aerobic and anaerobic bacteriology. Laryngoscope 89, 992-997.

4. Frederick J and Braude AI. 1974. Anaerobic infection of the
   paranasal sinuses. N.Engl.J.Med. 290, 135-137.

5. Lundberg C, Carenfelt C, Engqvist S and Nord C-E. 1979.
    Anaerobic bacteria in maxillary sinusitis. Scand.J.Infect.Dis.
    19, 74-76.

6. Ingham HR, Selkon JB and Roxby CM. 1977. Bacteriological study
    of otogenic cerebral abscesses: chemotherapeutic role of
    metronidazole. Br.Med.J. 2, 991-993.

7. Moloy PJ. 1982. Anaerobic mastoiditis: A report of two cases
    with complications. Laryngoscope 92, 1311-1315.

8. Lundberg C, Lonnroth J, Marklund G and Nord C-E. 1981.
    Tinidazole in the treatment of infections of the upper
    respiratory tract. Scand.J.Inf.Dis. 26, 130-134.

9. Thore M, Burman LG and Holm SE. 1982. Streptococcus pneumoniae
    and three species of anaerobic bacteria in experimental otitis
    media in guinea-pigs. J.Inf.Dis. 145: 822-828.

10. Holdeman LV, Cato EP, Moore WEC. (ed.). Anaerobe laboratory
    manual 4th ed. Virginia Polytechnic Institute and State
    University, Blacksburg, 1977, 152 p.

11. Fulghum RS, Brinn JE, Smith AM, Daniel III HJ and Loesche PJ.
    1982. Experimental otitis media in gerbils and chinchillas with
    Streptococcus pneumoniae, Haemophilus influenzae and other
    aerobic and anaerobic bacteria. Infection and Immunity, 36,
    802-810.

12. Friedmann I. 1955. The comparative pathology of otitis media
    experimental and human. I. Experimental otitis of the
    guinea-pig. J.Laryngol.Otol. 69, 27-50.

13. Giebink GS, Payne EE, Mills EL, Juhn SK and Quie PG. 1976.
    Experimental otitis media due to Streptococcus pneumoniae.
    Immunopathogenic response in the chinchilla. J.Infect.Dis. 134,
    595-604.

14. Lewis DM, Schram JL, Meadema SJ and Lim DJ. 1980. Experimental
    otitis media in chinchillas. Ann.Otol.Rhinol.Laryngol. 89,
    344-350.

SUCCESS AND FAILURE IN THE ASSOCIATION OF ANAEROBES FROM HUMAN
SUBGINGIVAL PLAQUE WITH CONVENTIONAL AND GNOTOBIOTIC RATS

B. GUGGENHEIM, R. GMUR AND C. WYSS

1. INTRODUCTION

The concept that bacteria are a prime factor in the aetiology of
periodontal disease has prevailed during the last twenty years
(1,2). Consequently the microbial composition of the subgingival
pocket flora was carefully analysed, using refined anaerobic culture
techniques (3,4) and by direct examination with darkfield-microscopy
(5). As a result of these efforts the so called specific plaque
hypothesis gained credibility, postulating the association of
distinct sets of Gram-negative anaerobes with clinically distinct
forms of periodontal disease. Among the bacteria thus implicated
are Actinobacillus actinomycetemcomitans (A. ac.) in localized
juvenile periodontitis and motile rods, spirochetes and the black
pigmented Bacteroides gingivalis (B. gingivalis) and Bacteroides
melaninogenicus intermedius (B. mel. intermedius) in several forms
of adult periodontitis (6,7,8,9).

In hamsters and rats, periodontal disease was demonstrated to be
transmissible with Actinomyces viscosus (A. viscosus) as the
aetiologic agent (10,11). In man, however, Actinomyces species were
found to be associated with gingivitis and root caries but not with
periodontitis (12,13). In view of these findings, it seemed
reasonable to attempt to increase the fidelity of the
A. viscosus-based animal model by trying to associate gnotobiotic
and conventional rats with microorganisms isolated from human
periodontal pockets. Since the basic studies of Gibbons, Socransky
and Kapsimalis in 1964 (14), in particular, the establishment of
human strains of pigmented Bacteroides in rodents has been
considered to be most difficult if not impossible. In particular,
the monoassociation of germfree rats with black pigmented
Bacteroides strains appeared to be almost a programmed failure.

However, superinfection of animals previously monoassociated with
A. viscosus seemed to be more promising. In the present paper we
describe experimental conditions which led to the successful
association of several Gram-negative anaerobes originating from
human periodontal pockets with gnotobiotic and conventional rats.

2. MATERIAL AND METHODS

Culture conditions. Wilkins Chalgren anaerobe agar (Oxoid)
supplemented with 5% (v/v) haemolyzed human blood was used as solid
medium for Bacteroides and Fusobacterium strains. A. viscosus Ny 1
was grown in Actinomyces broth (Difco). A. ac. A370 was cultured on
brain heart infusion agar (Difco). Treponema denticola CD 1
(T. denticola) was grown on a solid or fluid medium devised by
Dr. Barbara Laughton (Boston, Ma.). For fluid cultures, all
bacteria except T. denticola and A. viscosus were grown in a
modification (15) of a fluid medium (FUM) originally described by
Loesche et al. (16). Cultures of A. ac. and A. viscosus were
incubated at $37^{\circ}C$ in an atmosphere of 10% CO_2 in air. The other
bacteria were incubated at $37^{\circ}C$ in anaerobic jars (Baltimore
Biochemical Laboratories).

The ability of all strains to grow in a water extract of diet
2000 (see below) was investigated. To this end one part of sucrose
free diet was extracted with two parts of water (w/w) by stirring
overnight. The solids were removed by centrifugation and filtration
and the extract was finally filter-sterilized.

Experimental arrangements in rat studies. In the three
experiments described herein inbred RIC (rat inbred at Carworth
Farm, New York, N.Y.)-Sprague Dawley rats, obtained from the Roche
Institute fur Medizinisch-Biologische Forschung AG, Fullinsdorf,
Switzerland, were used.

The animals received the following three diets as indicated in
the experimental protocol: (i) powder-diet 2000S, containing 56%
sucrose, 5% wheat flour, 28% skim milk powder, 3% Arabon (Nestle),
2.5% dried yeast, 2.5% yeast extract (Oxoid), 2% geveral protein

(Lederle), 1% NaCl and a supplement according to Gustafsson's diet D 7 (17). (ii) diet 2000M, differing from diet 2000S in that it contained 60% wheat flour and only 1% sucrose. (iii) highly vitamized stock-diet 857 from Nafag, Gossau, Switzerland. Tap water and diet were available ad libitum. For the gnotobiotic experiment the diets were sterilized by gamma-irradiation (3Mrad) and the water was autoclaved. Housing of the animals, isolators and other general procedures have been previously described (18,19). Alveolar bone loss was measured by a radiographic method (20).

Experiment 1: The outline of the gnotobiotic experiment is shown in Fig. 1. At the average age of 28 days, 45 animals from four litters were divided into three sex and litter matched groups and were transferred to three isolators.

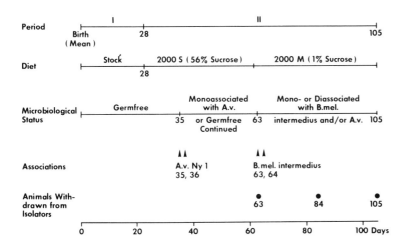

Fig. 1 Outline of the experiment with gnotobiotic rats.

Up to this time point, the rats were fed with stock-diet. From day 28 to day 63 the rats received diet 2000S. On days 35 and 36 the animals of two isolators were associated with A. viscosus while

those in the third isolator remained germfree. During the evening
of day 62, diet 2000S was replaced in all three isolators by diet
2000M. On days 63 and 64, the rats in the germfree isolator and in
one of the two other isolators were four times associated with
10^7-10^8 viable cells of B. mel. intermedius OMZ 248. Three and
four animals respectively, were withdrawn from each isolator and
decapitated, while the remaining eight animals were sacrificed at
the end of the experiment on day 105.

Experiment 2: In a second trial, conventional rats were used to
attempt the establishment of B. mel. intermedius. The experiment
consisted of three treatments, all with eight animals from three
litters. All animals were associated with A. viscous at the age of
30 days and treated from day 57 to 59 with kanamycin (10 mg/1) and
vanomycin (75 mg/1). On days 59 and 60 one group was associated
with B. mel. intermedius OMZ 248, while a second received another
B. mel. intermedius strain (OMZ 245) isolated from a case of rapidly
progressing periodontitis. All other experimental conditions were
as described for the gnotobiotic experiment, except that the
experimental period was prolonged to day 143 and that four animals
from each treatment were sacrificed on day 101.

Experiment 3: Table 6 provides the outline of this trial. Four
groups of 8 conventional rats (I-IV) were superinfected with
A. viscous and 3 anaerobes in different combinations. The
experiment lasted 164 days. The first four animals from each group
were sacrificed on day 115. All other conditions were as described
in experiment 2.

Confirmation of the establishment of bacteria in the oral cavity
of experimental rats. During these experiments, several techniques
were evaluated to monitor the establishment of bacteria in the oral
cavity of the animals:
(i) Post mortem samples taken with a miniloop from the gingival
margin were streaked on suitable selective media. (ii) Oral
swabbings collected from living animals were transferred to
selective media and further diluted using the streak-plate technique.

Alternatively, the material on the cotton of the applicator stick
was smeared on to a glass slide. After heat fixation, the bacteria
on the slide were stained with fluorescence labelled rabbit
antibodies specific for the associated bacteria. (iii) Maxillae and
mandibulae were excised immediately after decapitation and pressed
onto suitable solid selective media. The imprint formed a coarse
negative replica of the molar teeth and the gingival margin. (iv)
The excised jaws were placed on a precooled (approx. 8°C) layer of
Wilkins Chalgren blood agar and were then completely embedded with
the same agar medium without blood. Whenever the establishment of
Bacteroides strains was investigated the embedding medium further
contained 0.1 mg/l kanamycin and 7.5 mg/l vanomycin. The medium for
T. denticola was supplemented with 50 mg/l rifampicin. For
Fusobacterium a selective solid medium described by Walker et al.
(21) was used.

3. RESULTS

Growth of bacteria on diet extract in dependance of sucrose
concentration. In the experiment shown in Table 1 strains of
B. asaccharolyticus, B. mel. intermedium, A. viscosus, but not A.
ac. were able to grow in the fluid media. However, limited or no
growth of black pigmented strains was observed at sucrose
concentrations of 5% and more. In contrast, on solid medium the
growth limiting sucrose concentration for the black pigmenting
strains was around 10%. A. ac. showed ample growth at this
concentration. A. viscosus grew abundantly on fluid and solid media
at all sucrose concentrations tested.

Table 1 Growth of bacteria on solid and fluid diet extract
containing varying amounts of sucrose.

Sucrose Content %	Fluid medium*					Solid medium**				
	0	1	5	10	20	0	1	5	10	20
B. asaccharolyticus NCTC 9337	++	++	+	+	+−	++	++	++	+−	−
B. mel. intermedius UJB-13c	++	++	−	−	−	++	++	++	+−	+−
A. actinomycetem-comitans A 370	−	−	−	−	−	−	++	++	++	−
A. viscosus Ny 1	++	++	++	++	++	++	++	++	++	++

++ abundant growth   + limited growth   +− trace of growth   *72 h   **6 days

In the following, we investigated the growth of a number of
potentially pathogenic anaerobes in prereduced fluid diet extract
containing 1% sucrose with and without 5% heat-inactivated rat
serum. These results are compiled in Table 2.

Table 2 Growth of potentially pathogenic anaerobes in pre-reduced
fluid diet extract containing 1% sucrose with and without
5% inactivated rat serum.

	Growth without Serum	Growth with Serum
Bacteroides gingivalis W 1	+	++
Bacteroides gingivalis 381	−	++
Bacteroides gingivalis 10-2-1	−	++
B. mel. melaninogenicus OMZ 255	++	++
B. mel. intermedius OMZ 248	++	n. d.
Fusobacterium nucleatum OMZ 274	++	++
Treponema denticola CD 1	−	−

N = 3   − = no growth   + = limited growth   ++ = abundant growth
n.d. = not determined

Strains of B. mel. melaninogenicus, B. mel. intermedius, and
Fusobacterium nucleatum (F. nucleatum) showed ample growth in the
medium without serum. Strains of B. gingivalis grew poorly or not
at all. The addition of 5% rat serum which mimics to some extent
crevicular transudate or exudate in the oral cavity resulted in
proliferation of all strains of B. gingivalis. T. denticola CD 1
could not be cultured with or without serum. Since we intended to
associate T. denticola, we preincubated the diet-extract-medium with
a number of strains, and added 10% of the thus conditioned medium to
fresh medium to investigate the effect on the growth of T. denticola.
As shown in Table 3 the culture supernatants of A. viscosus and A.
ac. had no effect, while all media conditioned by black pigmenting
strains were growth promoting. A very strong growth promoting
effect was evident when supernatants of the asaccharolytic species
B. asaccharolyticus and B. gingivalis were added.

As a consequence of these experiments diet 2000M containing 1%
sucrose was selected for use whenever strains of these Gram-negative
anaerobes were to be associated with rats.

Table 3   Growth of T. denticola in prereduced, fluid diet extract
          containing 1% sucrose, 5% inactivated rat serum and 10% of
          various culture supernatants.

Origin of Supernatant	Growth
A. viscosus Ny 1	−
B. asaccharolyticus NCTC 9337	++
B. mel. melaninogenicus OMZ 255	+
B. gingivalis W 1	++
B. gingivalis 381	++
B. gingivalis 10-2-1	++
Fusobact. nucleatum OMZ 274	+
Actinobact. actinomycetemcomitans A 370	−

N = 3   − = no growth   + = limited growth   ++ = abundant growth

58

Viability of bacteria used for association with animals. In
order to ensure that the bacteria used for association were in an
optimum condition, the viability of these anaerobes was studied as a
function of the incubation time and of the time of exposure to air
necessary to prepare the inocula. Fluid cultures incubated for 24
to 96 hours were centrifuged, resuspended in reduced medium, and
exposed to air for 25, 90, and 180 minutes at room temperature. A
series of dilutions were prepared, plated on suitable solid media
and incubated anaerobically. It is evident from Fig. 2 that an
exposure to air of up to 180 minutes did not decrease the viability
of these anaerobes. Fig. 2 also shows that for B. gingivalis and
F. nucleatum the length of the incubation time did not appear to be
critical, while B. mel. intermedius exhibited a sharp decrease in
viability when cultures were incubated longer than 24 h. Similar
experiments with T. denticola CD 1 showed that cells intended for
association were best incubated for 72 to 120 h. An exposure to air
of up to 90 min in the reduced medium did not decrease the viability
significantly.

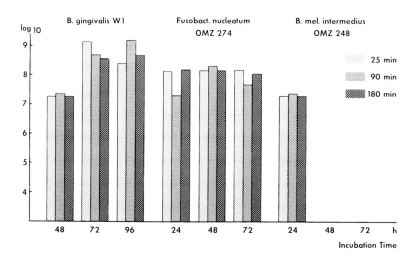

Fig. 2 Viability of bacteria in function of incubation time and of
time of exposure to air.

Animal experiments. Experiment 1: A. viscosus formed massive supragingival plaque and could be reisolated from all animals using the loop technique (data not shown). B. mel. intermedius OMZ 248 could only be reisolated with the novel impression technique. Both monoassociated and diassociated animals harboured the organism 21 days after the association, but only in the diassociated rats did the infection persist for 42 days (Table 4). Fig. 3A shows the culture of an impression replica, demonstrating that the organism was present along the gingival margin.

Table 4 Reisolation of B. mel. intermedius from gnotobiotic rats.

Treatment	Age of Animals Days	Days after Association with OMZ 248	Positive Loop Samples	Positive Replica
Monoassociated with B.mel. OMZ 248	84 105	21 42	0/3 0/7	2/3 0/7
Diassociated with OMZ 248 and Ny 1	84 105	21 42	0/3 0/7	2/3 6/7
Monoassociated with Ny 1	84 105	21 42	0/3 0/7	n.d. n.d.

Fig. 4 shows the degree of bone loss in the animals. A significant difference (p 0.01) was found for the groups mono- or diassociated with A. viscosus versus the group monoassociated with B. mel intermedius. The alveolar bone loss in the group monoassociated with B. mel. intermedius OMZ 248 was comparable with that of germfree animals (19).

Experiment 2:, In this trial using conventional animals experimentally associated with A. viscosus Ny 1 the establishment of the B. mel. intermedius strains OMZ 248 and 245 could be followed more closely. Bacteroides could not be detected one day after the association, but was consistantly present thereafter as shown by, at least, one technique during a period covering 85 days (Table 5).

Cells of B. mel. intermedius were found on the distal slopes of the rugae of the hard palate, on the soft palatinal mucosa, on the buccal vestibular mucosa, and along the gingival margin (Fig. 3B).

Fig. 3 Colonies of B. mel. intermedius growing along the impression of a jaw imprint (A) and within the selective medium in which a maxillae had been embedded (B)

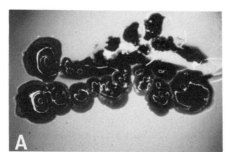
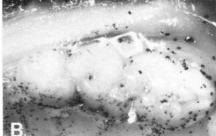

Table 5 Confirmation of the establishment of B. mel. intermedius strains in conventional rats.

	Age of Rats Days	Days after Association with Bacteroides	Positive Swab-Cultures	Positive Fluorescence	Positive Embedding Technique
	59	1	n.d.	0/8	n.d.
	70	12	4/4	3/4	n.d.
Infection	77	19	4/4	4/4	n.d.
with Ny 1	84	26	4/4	1/4	n.d.
and OMZ 248	98	40 *	2/3	0/3	3/3
	114	56	4/4	n.d.	n.d.
	121	63	2/2	2/2	n.d.
	143	85 *	2/3	n.d.	3/3
	59	1	n.d.	0/8	n.d.
	70	12	3/4	3/4	n.d.
Infection	77	19	4/4	3/3	n.d.
with Ny 1	84	26	4/4	4/4	n.d.
and OMZ 245	98	40	1/2	0/2	2/2
	114	56	4/4	n.d.	n.d.
	121	63	2/2	2/2	n.d.
	143	85	0/3	n.d.	3/3

Although none of these methods is quantitative, the results
suggest that the level of colonization fluctuated, reaching peak
levels 63 days after inoculation. Forty days after the association
a rather low degree of colonization was evident. Although the post
mortem embedding technique demonstrated that B. mel. intermedius OMZ
248 persisted in all animals, only 2 out of 3 rats showed a positive
swab culture (asterisk in Table 5) and all of them were negative if
judged by immunofluorescence. Finally, at the end of the
experiment, the colonization had again reached such low levels that
B. mel. intermedius OMZ 248 could only be demonstrated by the
embedding technique.

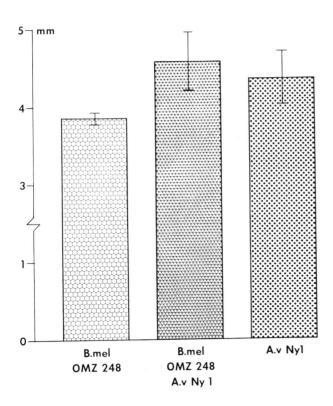

Fig 4   Mandibular bone loss in rats mono- or diassociated with
A. viscosus Ny 1 and B. mel. intermedius OMZ 248 (N = 8 per
treatment).

Bone loss in all three experimental groups was similar indicating that B. mel. intermedius had no significant effect.

Experiment 3: As indicated in Table 6 only A. viscosus persisted during the entire experimental period. All other strains either did not colonize or were gradually eliminated. B. gingivalis could only be detected occasionally in treatment II, III, and IV. In contrast, the colonization with F. nucleatum of the oral cavity of all animals of groups III and IV was demonstrated up to 42 days after the last association by positive swab cultures on the selective CVE agar and by positive immunofluorescence. Surprisingly, however, this strain was totally eliminated from the oral flora of all rats by day 164.

The colonization with T. denticola CD 1 of most animals of group IV was demonstrated on days 83 and 90 by phase-contrast and immunofluorescence-microscopy and on day 115 by the embedding technique. However, on day 164 T. denticola could no longer be detected in any of these animals (N = 4). No significant difference in the amount of alveolar bone loss between the four groups was observed.

Table 6   Outline of an experiment with conventional rats in which the
association of several potentially pathogenic human
anaerobes was attempted (N = 8 per treatment).

Treatment		Age of Animals at which Infection was Attempted	Number of Associations	Persistence of Infection
I	A. viscosus Ny 1	37, 38	4	+
II	A. viscosus Ny 1	37, 38	4	+
	+ B. gingivalis W 1	65, 66, 72, 73	8	−
III	A. viscosus Ny 1	37, 38	4	+
	− B. gingivalis W 1	65, 66, 72, 73	8	−
	+ Fusobact. nucleatum OMZ 274	65, 66, 72, 73	8	+
IV	A. viscosus Ny 1	37, 38	4	+
	+ B. gingivalis W 1	65, 66, 72, 73	8	−
	+ Fusobact. nucleatum OMZ 274	65, 66, 72, 73	8	−
	+ Treponema denticola CD 1	79, 80, 86, 87	8	−

4. DISCUSSION

The establishment of anaerobes originating from human
periodontal pockets in the oral cavity of rats depends on a number
of factors: (i) The presence of ecological niches allowing the
adsorbtion and growth of these microorganisms. These niches need
not primarily be located in the oral cavity, since a translocation
of bacteria may occur if the gingival conditions are modified by
e.g. a marginal inflammation. In the experiments described here, we
decided to create gingivitis by associating our rats with
A. viscosus Ny 1 prior to the infection with anaerobes. This strain
gives rise to ample supragingival plaque, provoking a strong local
inflammatory reaction. A permanent association of B. mel.
intermedius with gnotobiotic rats was only achieved under these
conditions. (ii) A diet for the animals which contains no
components inhibitory for the anaerobes to be associated but enables
these bacteria to grow, possibly with the help of host derived
nutrients, or with the help of growth factors produced by the
accompanying flora. In the present study, we have shown that black
pigmenting Bacteroides strains were sensitive to sucrose. This led
to the modification of diet 2000S replacing 55% sucrose by wheat
flour. In spite of a reduced sucrose content in the diet extract,
the growth of B. gingivalis was dependent on the addition of 5% rat

serum, while <u>T. denticola</u> furthermore needed growth factors efficiently produced by asaccharolytic <u>Bacteroides</u> strains. Most probably these growth factors are volatile acids as shown by Socransky <u>et al</u> (22). (iii) The number and the vability of the anaerobes used for association of experimental animals. The techniques described in this paper allowed the preparation of bacterial suspensions to inoculate at least 10^7 viable cells per rat. Not directly related, but of equal importance was the development of techniques which allowed a confirmation of the establishment of the associated bacteria in the oral cavity of the rats. Techniques commonly used to reisolate supragingival plaque bacteria (loop technique, oral swabs), as well as immunofluorescence were shown to be less sensitive than the newly developed replica technique. The best results were obtained with the technique of embedding entire jaws in selective media. (iv) Specific or unspecific host defense mechanisms which are naturally present or which build up in the animals after association with the bacteria. These factors are important, but hardly controllable. (v) Interactions of bacteria in the animals. This is in particularly important when conventional rats are used.

One or more of these factors were most probably responsible for the total failure to associate <u>B. gingivalis</u> and for the elimination of <u>F. nucleatum</u> and <u>T. denticola</u> from the oral cavity of the rats in experiment 3. The fact that a <u>Treponema</u> species could be associated, for as short a period as 24 days, with rats has not been previously reported. These experiments are a promising start to elucidate, in an animal model, the role of these and other anaerobes isolated from human periodontal diseases.

In future experiments the high pathogenicity of <u>A. viscosus</u> Ny1 must be considered. This strain is able to produce periodontal bone loss when monoassociated with germfree animals or superinfected in conventional rats. Ideally, the strain should be replaced by a supragingival plaque forming organism which causes a gingival inflammation but no alveolar bone loss. The pathogenicity of <u>A. viscosus</u> Ny 1 may have obscured a potential pathogenic effect of the anaerobes. This is suspected, particularly, for <u>B. mel. intermedius</u> OMZ 248, since we have shown earlier that it invades the periodontal connective tissue in gnotobiotic rats (23).

REFERENCES

1. Van Palenstein Helderman WH. 1981. Microbial etiology of periodontal disease. J. Clin. Periodontol. 8: 261-280.
2. Slots J. 1979. Subgingival microflora and periodontal disease. J. Clin. Periodontol. 6: 351-382.
3. Tanner ACR, Haffer C, Bratthal FT, Visconti RA, Socransky SS. 1979. A study of the bacteria associated with advancing periodontitis in man. J. Clin. Periodontol. 6: 278-307.
4. Moore WEC, Holdeman LV, Smibert RM, Hash DE, Burgmeister JA, Ranney RR. 1982. Bacteriology of severe periodontitis in young adult humans. Infection and Immunity 38: 1137-1148.
5. Listgarten MA, Hellden L. 1978. Relative distribution of bacteria at clinically healthy and periodontally diseased sites in human. J. Clin. Periodontol. 5: 115-132.
6. Newman MG. 1979. The role of Bacteroides melaninogenicus and other anaerobes in periodontal infections. Rev. Infect. Dis. 1: 313-323.
7. White D, Mayrand D. 1981. Association of oral Bacteroides with gingivitis and adult periodontitis. J. Periodontal Res. 16: 259-265.
8. Zambon JJ, Reynolds HS, Slots J. 1981. Black-pigmented Bacteroides spp. in the human oral cavity. Infect. Immun. 32: 198-203.
9. Listgarten MA, Levin S. 1981. Positive correlation between the proportions of subgingival spirochetes and motile bacteria and susceptibility of human subjects to periodontal deterioration. J. Clin. Periodontol. 8: 122-138.
10. Jordan HV, Fitzgerald RJ, Stanley HR 1965. Plaque formation and periodontal pathology in gnotobiotic rats infected with an oral actinomycete. Am. J. Pathol. 47: 1157-1167.
11. Georg LK, Pine L, Gerencer MA. 1969. Actinomyces viscosus, comb. nov., a catalase positive, facultative member of the genus Actinomyces. Int. J. Syst. Bact. 19: 291-293.
12. Loesche WJ, Syed SA. 1978. Bacteriology of human experimental gingivitis: effect of plaque and gingivitis score. Infect. Immun. 21: 830-839.
13. Jordan HV, Sumney DL. 1973. Root-surface caries: review of the literature and significance of the problem. J. Periodontol. 44: 158-163.
14. Gibbons RJ, Socransky SS, Kapsimalis B. 1964. Establishment of human indigenous bacteria in germ-free mice. J. Bacteriol. 88: 1316-1323.
15. Gmur R, Guggenheim B. 1983. Antigenic heterogeneity of Bacteroides intermedius as recognized by monoclonal antibodies. Infect. Immun. 42: in press.
16. Loesche WJ, Hockett RN, Syed SA. 1972. The predominant cultivable flora of tooth surface plaque removed from institutionalized subjects. Archs oral Biol. 17: 1311-1325.
17. Luckey TD. 1963. Germfree life and gnotobiology. New York Academic Press Inc., p. 494.
18. Guggenheim B, Schroeder HE. 1974. Reactions in the periodontium to continuous antigenic stimulation in sensitized gnotobiotic rats. Infect. Immun. 10: 565-577.

66

19. Burckhardt JJ, Gaegauf-Zollinger R, Schmid R, Guggenheim B. 1981. Alveolar bone loss in rats after immunization with Actinomyces viscosus. Infect. Immun. 31: 971-977.
20. Gaegauf-Zollinger R, Burckhardt JJ, Guggenheim B. 1982. Radiographic measurements of alveolar bone loss in the rat. Archs oral Biol. 27: 651-658.
21. Walker CB, Ratliff D, Muller C, Mandell R, Socransky SS. 1979. Medium for selective isolation of Fusobacterium nucleatum from human periodontal pockets. J. Clin. Microbiol. 10: 844-849.
22. Socransky SS, Loesche WJ, Hubersak C, MacDonald JB. 1964. Dependency of Treponema microdentium on other oral organisms for isobutyrate, polyamines, and a controlled oxidation-reduction potential. J. Bact. 88: 200-209.
23. Allenspach-Petrzilka GE, Guggenheim B. 1982. Bacteroides melaninogenicus ss. intermedium invasion of rat gingival tissue. J. Periodontal Res. 17: 456-459.

ENTEROCOLITIS OF PIGS

R.J. LYSONS

Swine dysentery, an infectious disease of pigs, in which the
lesions are confined to the large bowel, provides an interesting
example of the use of animal models in the study of an animal
disease. The most important model is the natural host itself, and
swine dysentery has been reproduced experimentally in conventional
pigs. In addition, other animal models of the disease have been
developed, namely the gnotobiotic pig (1), the guinea pig (2) and
the CFI mouse (3). The ligated colonic loop in pigs (4), though not
strictly an animal model, can be regarded as an _in vivo_ model.

This paper examines two aspects of swine dysentery research where
animal models can be of use. The first concerns attempts to identify
and define the role of the aetiological agents in swine dysentery.
The second is the study of the immunological response of the host in
this disease. The conventional pig, the gnotobiotic pig and the CF1
mouse, are the models of choice for purusing these two objectives.

Swine dysentery - the naturally occurring disease.

Swine dysentery characteristically affects pigs 3 to 10 weeks
after weaning. The animals develop diarrhoea containing mucus and
often blood. Dehydration is an early feature of the disease, seen
as a hollowing of the animals' flanks. Weight loss of progressive
and the animal becomes gaunt and weak. Up to 90% of animals may be
affected and 25% may die. Antibiotic therapy, given at any stage of
the disease, however, usually leads to rapid recovery. Swine
dysentery is widespread in the pig population and is largely
controlled by antibiotics, often given in the feed, continuously,
from weaning to slaughter.

The aetiological agents of swine dysentery.

The search for the causal agents of swine dysentery has been a
protracted one. The disease was first described in the USA by
Whiting, Doyle and Spray in 1921 (5). There were conflicting reports
in the 1940's and 1950's as to the role of Vibrio (Campylobacter)
coli. It was not until 1971 that two groups, working independently,
were able to demonstrate that cultures of a sphirochaete,
subsequently named Treponema hyodysenteriae, could reproduce the
disease when given as an oral dose (6,7).

For many years attempts to produce the disease with pure cultures
of T. hyodysenteriae in gnotobiotic pigs were unsuccessful. Meyer
et al (1), using a combination of T. hyodysenteriae and 4 other
anaerobes, were eventually able to produce a mild colitis.

The implication was that T. hyodysenteriae acted synergistically
with other agents to produce the lesions. Attempts to identify these
organisms were made by comparing the anaerobic flora associated with
the colonic mucosa in healthy pigs and in pigs with swine dysentery
(8-10). Bacteroides vulgatus and Fusobacterium necrophorum were
isolated in large numbers from experimentally-induced lesions of
swine dysentery in a hysterectomy-derived, colostrum-deprived pig.
Either of these organisms together with T. hyodysenteriae was able
to induce lesions in gnotobiotic pigs (11,12). Subsequently,
however, it was shown that any one of several different organisms in
combination with T. hyodysenteriae could produce similar lesions
(13).

The action of T. hyodysenteriae by itself in the gnotobiotic pig
could not be studied because attempts to establish the organism alone
in the colon were unsuccessful. Recently, however, workers in the
USA were able to demonstrate that T. hyodysenteriae could multiply
by itself in the colon of the gnotobiotic pig, and that lesions were
produced (14,15). This satisfied Koch's postulates, showing that T.
hyodysenteriae is a pathogen in its own right. The mild nature of
the disease in gnotobiotic pigs compared with acute swine dysentery
(Table 1) suggests that other organisms are involved in increasing
the severity of the disease.

TABLE 1   Animal models of T. hyodysenteriae infection

Animal model	Clinical disease	Gross pathology
Conventional pig	excretion of blood, mucus dehydration death	acute colitis
Gnotobiotic pig	excretion of mucus appetite unimpaired	mild colitis
CF1 mouse	no clinical disease	mild typhlitis

The role of T. hyodysenteriae in lesion production.

1. The conventional and hysterectomy-derived, colostrum-deprived
   pig   The disease experimentally produced in conventional pigs
   (Table 1 and Figure 1) is indistinguishable from that seen in
   natural outbreaks in the field.

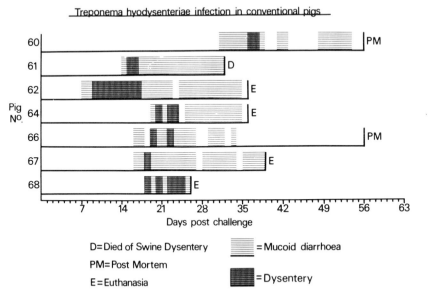

Treponema hyodysenteriae infection in conventional pigs

D = Died of Swine Dysentery   = Mucoid diarrhoea
PM = Post Mortem
E = Euthanasia   = Dysentery

The incubation period is relatively long and variable, usually 5 to 14 days, but sometimes it can be 28 days or longer. It has been difficult to produce early acute disease and to examine the initial pathological changes. It has been assumed that T. hyodysenteriae initiates the disease process and hence is responsible for the early lesions.

As methods for growing T. hyodysenteriae in broth have improved (16,17) it has been possible to dose pigs with larger numbers of actively motile organisms. The result of this has been to decrease the incubation period. In a recent experiment, hysterectomy-derived, colostrum-deprived (HDCD) pigs were given 2 oral inocula of T. hyodysenteriae totalling 5×10^{10} to 1×10^{11} organisms per animal (Lysons, Pohlenz, Harris and Whipp, unpublished). In a number of animals dysentery was observed 48 hours later. The animals were examined in the early stages of the disease, 8/10 were killed between 2 and 5 days after inoculation. In these early acute cases an intense reddening of the colonic mucosa was observed. In many pigs this extended from the tip of the caecum to the rectum. Mucus was present in the faeces and was observed as a thin layer covering the colonic mucosa, the contents in the lumen being fluid. In later stages of the disease mucus and fibrin formed a pseudomembrane over extensive areas of the mucosa and much of the contents of the colon consisted of mucus, fibrin, inflammatory cells and damaged epithelial cells. Swine dysentery is essentially a catarrhal enteritis, the lesion being one of a coagulative necrosis of the surface epithelial cells.

TABLE 2 Histopathology of lesions

	Conventional pig	Gnotobiotic pig	CF1 mouse
Hyperaemia	+++	+	±
Mucus release	+++	+++	++
Epithelial cell exfoliation	+++	+/++	+
Epithelial cell hyperplasia	+++	++	++
Inflammatory cell infiltration	+++	+/++	+

The main histopathological features of the colon and caecum of these early cases are summarised in Table 2, and may be recognised as being part of the naturally-occurring disease. The blood vessels of the mucosa and submucosa were greatly dilated. This hyperaemia would cause the dramatic reddening seen at post mortem examination. The colonic crypts were dilated with mucus and some mucus was seen on the surface. The majority of the goblet cells, particularly in the lower part of the crypt, had expressed their mucus. Surface epithelial cells had an abnormal appearance and there was exfoliation with small areas of erosion. A marked hyperplasia of epithelial cells could be recognised by the increased number of mitotic figures. Undifferentiated, immature epithelial cells lined the lower part of the crypt. There was a marked mononuclear and polymorphonuclear cell infiltration of the mucosa. In some pigs there was oedema of the lamina propria and submucosa. The lesions represented reaction of the animal to an intensely irritant effect which would have coincided with the presence of large numbers of T. hyodysenteriae in the caecum and colon. Spirochaetes could be seen deep in the crypts at this stage. The most striking effects were the massive release of mucus from goblet cells and the hyperplasia of epithelial cells. Both these phenomena could have been triggered off by epithelial cell damage.

The oral inoculation of gnotobiotic pigs and CFI mice with
T. hyodysenteriae did not result in disease identical with swine
dysentery, as can be seen from Table 1. They represent,
however, the effect of T. hyodysenteriae infection in these
animal models and were examined to assist the assessment of the
role of the spirochaete in early lesions.

2. The gnotobiotic pig As mentioned earlier, the clinical disease
   in gnotobiotic pigs is very mild (Table 1). Clinical signs and
   lesions in gnotobiotic pigs mono-associated with T.hyodysenteriae
   have been described (14,15). The histopathological features
   found in the conventional and HDCD pig are seen also in the
   gnotobiotic pig, but are less severe (Table 2). Expulsion of
   mucus from large numbers of goblet cells was observed in the
   early stages of the disease.
   Electron microscopic studies have revealed spirochaetes within
   goblet cells in 4 of 8 pigs inoculated with T. hyodysenteriae
   (15). There have been earlier reports of spirochaetes within
   goblet cells and damaged epithelial cells, but this consistent
   finding in gnotobiotic pigs suggests that the initial invasion
   of goblet cells may be the method of breaching the integrity of
   the surface of the large intestine.

3. The CF1 mouse Oral dosing of the CF1 mouse with cultures of T.
   hyodysenteriae results in a caecal infection and typhlitis (3).
   The lesions appear to be confined to the caecum and the gross
   appearance is of the caecum being filled (and sometimes
   distended) with mucus rather than the normal, semisolid,
   greenish contents. Detection of excess mucus in faeces is
   difficult and infected mice appear to suffer no ill effects.
   The histopathology again shows consistency of features with
   other animal models and the mouse would appear to be a useful
   model for studies of T. hyodysenteriae infection.
   If the evidence is correlated, it is possible to propose a
   sequence of events from the oral inoculation of T.
   hyodysenteriae to the development of lesions in the colon.

Spirochaetes have been seen in the bottom of colonic crypts 48 hours after inoculation. Their serpentine movement helps them to move through agar, and they are chemotactically attracted to substances in blood agar (Lysons, unpublished). It is likely that they are attracted to constituents of mucus and they move towards the surface of the colon and down the crypts. This may be the ecological niche of a number of the intestinal spirochaetes. Spirochaetes would follow the chemotactic gradient to its source, namely the goblet cell. Non-pathogenic variants of T. hyodysenteriae have been demonstrated inside goblet cells of gnotobiotic pigs (15). The pathogenic T. hyodysenteriae have the ability, perhaps through a toxin, to damage epithelial cells. There may even be a specific effect which results in goblet cell discharge. This would then allow more access of T. hyodysenteriae to the goblet cells.

Epithelial cell exfoliation has been demonstrated in gnotobiotic pigs inoculated with T. hyodysenteriae and either B. vulgatus or F. necrophorum (12). These small erosions in the conventional pig could be the site of entry of the other organisms which contribute to the lesion of swine dysentery.

Animal models of the immune response to T. hyodysenteriae. The immune response of animals to surface infections of the large intestine is, in general, poorly understood. What is apparent is that the pig can have difficulty in mounting an immune response sufficient to resolve the lesions of swine dysentery. Figure 1 shows that only 1 of 7 experimentally infected pigs managed to recover from the disease. Figure 2 shows that the CF1 mouse also has lesions which persist for several weeks (Lysons and Lemcke, unpublished). The mouse then could be a useful and very convenient model for studying the immune response of animals to T. hyodysenteriae. Two of the most pressing practical problems to be overcome in controlling swine dysentery could be helped by this fundamental knowledge. One is a need for sensitive and specific test for detecting pigs infected with T. hyodysenteriae; the other is the development of an effective vaccine for the disease.

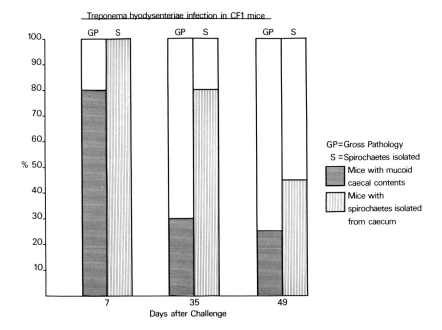

Treponema hyodysenteriae infection in CF1 mice

Conclusion

The development of animal models of swine dysentery has been achieved, but not without difficulty. It took 50 years from first recognition of the disease until its reproduction with T. hyodysenteriae in conventional pigs. Another 10 years elapsed before it was possible to demonstrate the pathogenicity of T. hyodysenteriae alone in the gnotobiotic pigs.

This paper has described how models can be and have been used to elucidate the role of aetiological agents of swine dysentery and also the immune response to large intestinal infections. Animal models other than the natural host have a limited usefulness. The gnotobiotic pig and the CF1 mouse may be valuable in studying T. hyodysenteriae infections but the diseases manifested are quite different from T. hyodysenteriae infection in the conventional pig. The only good model of swine dysentery is the conventional pig itself.

REFERENCES

1. Meyer RC, Simon J and Byerly CS. (1975). The etiology of swine dysentery. III. The role of selected Gram-negative obligate anaerobes. Veterinary Pathology 12, 46-56.
2. Joens LA, Songer JG, Harris DL and Glock RD. (1978). Experimental infection with Treponema hyodysenteriae in guinea pigs. Infection and Immunity 22, 132-135.
3. Joens LA and Glock RD. (1979). Experimental infection in mice with Treponema hyodysenteriae. Infection and Immunity 25, 757-760.
4. Whipp SC, Harris DL, Kinyon JM, Songer JG and Glock RD. (1978). Enteropathogenicity testing of Treponema hyodysenteriae in ligated colonic loops of swine. American Journal Veterinary Research 39, 1293-1296.
5. Whiting RA, Doyle LP and Spray RS. 1921). Swine dysentery. Purdue University Agricultural Experimental Station Bulletin 257, 1-15.
6. Taylor DJ and Alexander TJL. (1971). The production of dysentery in swine by feeding cultures containing a spirochaete. British Veterinary Journal 127, 58-61.
7. Harris DL, Glock RD, Christensen CR and Kinyon JM. (1972). Swine dysentery, 1. Inoculation of pigs with Treponema hyodysenteriae (new species) and reproduction of the disease. Veterinary Medicine and Small Animal Clinician 67, 61-64.
8. Alexander TJL and Wellstead PD. (1974). Bacteria isolated from scrapings of the mucosal wall of the colon. Proceedings 3rd Congress International Pig Veterinary Society, Abstract D 5.
9. Alexander TJL, Wellstead PD and Hudson MJ. (1976). Studies of bacteria other than Treponema hyodysenteriae which may contribute to the lesion of swine dysentery. Proceedings of the 4th Congress International Pig Veterinary Society, Abstract L1.
10. Robinson IM, Allison MJ and Whipp SC. (1982). Characterisation of bacteria adherent to colonic epithelia of pigs with dysentery. Proceedings Annual Meeting American Society for Microbiology, Abstract 158.
11. Harris DL, Alexander TJL, Whipp SC, Robinson IM, Glock RD and Matthews PJ. (1978). Swine dysentery: Studies of gnotobiotic pigs inoculated with Treponema hyodysenteriae, Bacteroides vulgatus and Fusobacterium necrophorum. Journal of the American Veterinary Medical Association 172, 468-471.
12. Lysons RJ, Hall GA, Alexander TJL, Bew J and Blanc AP. (1978). Aetiological agents and pathogenesis of swine dysentery. Proceedings 8th Congress International Pig Veterinary Society, Abstract M1.
13. Whipp SC, Robinson IM, Harris DL, Glock RD and Matthews PJ. (1980). Inoculation of gnotobiotic pigs with Treponema hyodysenteriae in the presence and absence of selected anaerobes. Proceedings 6th International Congress International Pig Veterinary Society p230.
14. Whipp SC, Pohlenz JFL, Harris DL, Robinson IM, Glock RD, Kunkle R. (1982). Pathogenicity of Treponema hyodysenteriae in uncontaminated gnotobiotic pigs. Proceedings 7th Congress International Pig Veterinary Society p31.

15. Pohlenz JFL, Lysons RJ, Whipp SC, Harris DL and Fargerland JA. (1983). Morphology of the intestinal mucosa in gnotobiotic pigs experimentally infected with a pathogenic and an apathogenic strain of <u>Treponema hyodysenteriae</u>. Proceedings 3rd International Symposium of Veterinary Laboratory Diagnosticians, p553-558.
16. Lemcke RM, Bew J, Burrows MR and Lysons RJ. (1979). The growth of <u>Treponema hyodysenteriae</u> and other porcine intestinal spirochaetes in a liquid medium. Research in Veterinary Science <u>26</u>, 315-319.

ANIMAL MODELS OF CLOSTRIDIUM SPIROFORME MEDIATED DIARRHOEA (IOTA
ENTEROTOXAEMIA) OF RABBITS

R.J. CARMAN AND S.P. BORRIELLO

1.   INTRODUCTION

In the late 1970s and early 1980s there were several reports of
a fatal diarrhoea of weaned rabbits (1-6). The features of the
disease were the demonstration in the caeca of dead animals of a
neutralizable iota-like toxin but the absence of detectable
Clostridium perfringens Type E, which is known to produce iota
toxin. It is now known that the causal organism is C. spiroforme
(7-9). In the light of current knowledge, samples from all but one
of the earlier outbreaks have been retrospectively analyzed and
shown to contain C. spiroforme and its toxin. The condition,
previously known as iota enterotoxaemia, can now be better termed
C. spiroforme mediated diarrhoea (SMD).

C. spiroforme is a semicircular organism which often forms
loosely coiled chains when it is grown in vitro (10). The organism
was first described by Kaneuchi et al (11) who collected isolates
from healthy adult humans and chickens, none of whom had a history
of diarrhoea or antimicrobial therapy. However, none of the
available isolates was able to produce iota-like toxin (R.J. Carman,
unpublished observation).

SMD has been induced in adult rabbits following challenge with clindamycin (12), lincomycin (6) and metronidazole (R.J. Carman, unpublished observation). Spontaneous disease, not only occurs in the European rabbit, Oryctolagus cuniculur (9) but also in eastern cotton-tail rabbits (J. Cary & R.H. Evans, personal communication). To date the spontaneous condition seems to be confined to lagomorphs. Recent work has shown that the disease is due to acquisition of C. spiroforme by an animal susceptible to colonisation due to antibiotic or weaning-induced disturbances of the gastrointestinal flora. This conclusion is based on the observations that, if adult animals are housed in isolators, both antibiotic and C. spiroforme must be administered to induce disease, neither alone being sufficient. In addition, newly weaned rabbits only succumbed to disease if first challenged with the organism (14). In order to study the epidemiology and pathogenesis of this disease it is necessary, in many cases, to house susceptible animals in flexible film isolators to prevent chance infection. However the costs and problems inherent in this procedure prompted us to investigate the possibility of using smaller and more easily managed laboratory animals. The search for alternative models was broadened when curved Gram positive rods, resembling C. spiroforme, were identified in non-mammalian animals such as chickens (11), turkeys (15) and leopard frogs (16).

2. MATERIALS AND METHODS

Animals

The following animals were used for these investigations:
New Zealand white and cross lop rabbits, Duncan Hartley guinea pigs, golden Syrian hamsters, WAG rats, CBA/CA mice, white leghorn chickens and Xenopus laevii toads. All animals received an antibiotic free diet ad libitum.

Organism

C. spiroforme NCTC 11493, an iota-like toxigenic bacterium isolated from a diarrhoeic rabbit was cultured on sheep blood agar for 48 h under anaerobic incubation conditions. Bacteria were harvested into sterile phosphate buffered saline to provide oral inocula of 10^5 organisms/ml. Inocula (1ml) were administered by a flexible rubber oral dosing tube.

Clindamycin

Animals were isolated in either clean rooms or isolators not previously used to house animals receiving clindamycin or C. spiroforme. Test animals were each given 3 successive daily i.p. doses of clindamycin, 15mg/kg/day. Thereafter, isolation or quarantine was maintained for 7 days before animals were dosed with C. spiroforme.

Experimental groups

In earlier work (14) it was established that clindamycin alone and C. spiroforme alone were both unable to elicit SMD. Only the disruption of the intestinal flora, either by clindamycin or by weaning, acting in consort with C. spiroforme could lead to SMD. Consequently, the experimental groups needed to consist of animals challenged with clindamycin alone or together with C. spiroforme. For every species of laboratory animal investigated 10 animals, 5 in either group, were studied.

Diagnosis of SMD

Animals receiving clindamycin alone were culled 14 days after the final i.p. challenge. They received a full post mortem examination. Caecal content from each was analyzed for the presence

of C. spiroforme using an alcohol wash technique for the selection
of sporulating clostridia (16). Iota-like toxin was assayed using
the mouse lethality, the guinea pig dermonecrosis assays (17) or
cytotoxicity in tissue culture (10). Animals dying with or culled
whilst suffering from diarrhoea were similarly investigated.

3. RESULTS

The results are presented in table 1.

Table 1. Susceptibility of various animal species to experimentally
induced C. spiroforme mediated diarrhoea

| | | Detection of | |
Animal	Disease	C. spiroforme	Toxin
Rabbit	+	+	+
Guinea pig	+	+	+
Syrian hamster	+	+	+
Rat	+	+	+
Mouse	+	+	+
Chicken	-	-	-
Toad	-	-	-

+ = Present;   - = Absent.

Rabbits, guinea pigs, hamsters and mice

Animals receiving only clindamycin showed no signs of SMD.
Neither C. spiroforme nor its toxin was detected. Conversely, all
those animals challenged with both clindamycin and C. spiroforme
became diarrhoeic and either died or became moribund and were
culled. Signs of diarrhoea first appeared often within 24 h, but
never later than 3 days, after challenge with C. spiroforme. From
the caeca of all diarrhoeic animals both C. spiroforme and its
iota-like toxin were detected. At no time was C. difficile or its
cytotoxin demonstrable.

Chickens and Xenopus laevii

Regardless of whether they received clindamycin alone or with organism, none of the chickens or toads exhibited signs of SMD. C. spiroforme was not recovered from the guts of these animals.

4   DISCUSSION

The induction of classical SMD in rabbits has already been demonstrated (9, 12, 14, 18). The current report is the first description of the condition in animals other than lagomorphs. These observations broaden the range of potential models for the study of SMD in species more easily and more cheaply managed in flexible film isolators. It must be stressed that isolation techniques are essential for the satisfactory investigation of SMD. For example, three guinea pigs given a single dose of clindamycin, were moved to cages besides diarrhoeic rabbits; all succumbed to SMD within 72h. That animals other than lagomorphs are prone to infection, albeit under experimental conditions, provides support for the possibility that C. spiroforme could be associated with gastrointestinal disorders in man. Furthermore, it infers that consideration of C. spiroforme as an alternative cause of diarrhoea is necessary in research into antibiotic associated colitis apparently mediated by C. difficile.

It is interesting that we were unable to produce disease in either chickens or toads. In respect to the latter it may be that as cold blooded animals the body temperature is inadequate for in vivo growth of the strain of C. spiroforme used. This possibility is supported by the fact that the organism fails to grow on agar plates when incubated at room temperature. Chickens may be insensitive to colonization for a variety of reasons, amongst which must be included the differences in anatomy and physiology of the avian and mammalian alimentary tracts.

REFERENCES

1. ORCUTT RP FOSTER HL JONAS AM. 1978. Clostridium perfringens
    Type E enterotoxaemia as the cause of acute diarrheal death or
    "hemorrhagic typhlitis" in rabbits. Amer. Assoc. Lab. Anim.
    Sci., Abstract 100 in publication 78-4.

2. PATTON NM HOLMES HT RIGGS RJ CHEEKE PR. 1978. Enterotoxemia
    in rabbits. Lab. Anim. Sci., 28, 536-540.

3. FERNIE DS EATON P. 1980. The demonstration of a toxin
    resembling Clostridium perfringens iota toxin in rabbits with
    enterotoxaemia. FEMS Microbiol. Letters, 8, 33-35.

4. EATON P FERNIE DS. 1980. Enterotoxaemia involving Clostridium
    perfringens iota toxin in a hysterectomy-derived rabbit
    colony. Lab. Anim., 14, 347-351.

5. BASKERVILLE M WOOD M SEAMER JH. 1980. Clostridium perfringens
    type E enterotoxaemia in rabbits. Vet. Rec., 107, 18-19.

6. REHG JE PAKES SP. 1982. Implication of Clostridium difficile
    and Clostridium perfringens iota toxins in experimental
    lincomycin-associated colitis of rabbits. Lab. Anim. Sci., 32,
    253-257.

7. CARMAN RJ BORRIELLO SP. 1982. Observation on an association
    between Clostridium spiroforme and Clostridium perfringens Type
    E iota enterotoxaemia in rabbits. Eur. J. Chemother.
    Antibiot., 2, 143-144.

8. CARMAN RJ BORRIELLO SP. 1982. Clostridium spiroforme isolated
    from rabbits with diarrhoea. Vet. Rec. 111, 461-462.

9. BORRIELLO SP CARMAN RJ. 1983. Association of toxigenic
    Clostridium spiroforme with iota toxin positive enterotoxaemia
    in rabbits. J. Clin. Microbiol., 17, 414-418.

10. CARMAN RJ BORRIELLO SP. 1983. Laboratory diagnosis of
    Clostridium spiroforme mediated diarrhoea (iota enterotoxaemia)
    of rabbits. Vet. Rec. 113, 184-185.

11. KANEUCHI C MIYAZATO T SHINJO T MITSUOKA T. 1979. Taxonomic
    study of helically coiled sporeforming anaerobes isolated from
    the intestines of humans and other animals: Clostridium
    cocleatum sp. nov. and Clostridium spiroforme sp. nov. Int. J.
    Syst. Bacteriol., 29, 1-12.

12. LAMONT JT, SONNENBLICK EB, ROTHMAN SW. 1979. Role of clostridial toxin in the pathogenesis of clindamycin colitis in rabbits. Gastroenterology, 76, 356-361.

13. CARMAN RJ, BORRIELLO SP. in press. Epidemiology of experimental Clostridium spiroforme mediated diarrhoea of rabbits. Infect. Immun.

14. BEDBURY HP, DUKE GE. 1983. Cecal microflora of turkeys fed low or high fiber diets: enumeration, identification, and determination of cellulolytic activity. Poultry Sci., 62, 675-682.

15. GOSSLING J, LOESCHE WJ, NACE GW. 1982. Large intestine bacteria of nonhibernating and hibernating leopard frogs (Rana pipiens), Appl. Environ. Microbiol., 44, 59-66.

16. KORANSKY JR, ALLEN SD, DOWELL Jr VR. 1978. Use of ethanol for selective isolation of sporeforming microorganisms. Appl. Environ. Microbiol., 35, 762-765.

17. STERNE M, BATTY I. 1975. Pathogenic Clostridia. London, Butterworths, 79-84.

18. KATZ L, LAMONT JT, TRIER JS, SONNENBLICK EB, ROTHMAN SW, BROITMAN SA, RIETH S. 1978. Experimental clindamycin-associated colitis in rabbits. Evidence for toxin-mediated mucosal damage. Gastroenterology, 74, 246-252.

OVINE FOOTROT: HISTOPATHOLOGY OF A SYNERGIC DISEASE

PAUL M. HINE

INTRODUCTION

Current research described here has involved a thorough study of the histopathology of ovine footrot and has revealed a few anomalies in the current theories on the mechanisms involved in this economically important infection. Despite all the work that has been carried out to date, the use of modern investigative techniques can reveal new facts, some of which can be integrated with established opinions. Others pose new problems and suggest further lines of research that would have to be carried out in order to provide effective methods for control and eradication of footrot.

The numbers of bacteria that can be isolated from cases of ovine footrot can be quite considerable, due to the fact that the hoof is constantly exposed to faecal and environmental contamination. By using a combination of bacterial isolation and induction of experimental disease, however, an aetiology for footrot has emerged over the years[1,7,13]. Unfortunately, not all groups of workers agree to the composition of this mixed infection.

There are two current points of view on the way in which this disease manifests itself[6,9]. To some research workers, footrot is a mixed bacterial invasion induced by environmental conditions combined with predisposition to the disease by other infections such as foot and mouth disease or contagious ecthyma. The majority of workers feel that footrot is a specific synergic disease involving the five organisms shown in Table 1.

TABLE 1   Bacteria implicated in ovine footrot

Synergic disease	Polymicrobial syndrome
Corynebacterium pyogenes	Corynebacterium pyogenes
Fusobacterium necrophorum	Fusobacterium necrophorum
Bacteroides nodosus	Bacteroides nodosus
Treponema penortha	Bacteroides sp.
Unidentified motile fusiform	Aerobic bacilli
	Clostridium perfringens A
	Staphylococcus aureus

The advantages of a synergic infection, as opposed to a mixed invasion, is that the bacteria involved may as individuals be either non-pathogenic or weak pathogens. However, when they combine as a synergic infection their pathogenic potential is increased as they can provide growth factors and protective agents to enhance colonisation and penetration of the host tissues[14,15].

Both the synergic and mixed infection hypotheses have demonstrated the role of the bacteria in footrot by isolating representative strains from the lesions, reapplying them to healthy feet as pure and mixed cultures and making observations on the possible development of a disease similar to true footrot. There has been no evidence to show that further factors or organisms are not involved. Previous research on the development of the lesion has been carried out by sampling both natural and experimental disease and examining the tissues by normal light microscopic histological methods. The bacteria involved have thus been identified by morphology alone[7,13].

Use of immunocytochemistry in the light and electron microscopes combined with ultrastructural studies can enhance our understanding of the way in which the disease develops. Thus, using both natrual and experimental infections, it has been possible to identify positively in vivo those organisms postulated to occur within the early stages of footrot and to follow the growth and invasion of these organisms throughout the development of the lesion. An experimental schedule was developed which involved histological studies on normal and pathological ovine hooves. The isolation and characterization of bacteria from natural infections, the production of an experimental model in sheep using these isolates and a comparison of natural and experimental infection demonstrated that the model was equivalent to the natural disease.

Initially for both light and electron microscopy, the staining
reactions, structure and serology of the bacterial isolates had to
be examined. The latter was especially important since the
immunocytochemical techniques to be used (fluorochrome and
peroxidase-labelled antibodies) would have to be specific for a
particular species of bacteria. Comparisons were then made of
normal and pathological specimens of both natural and experimental
disease using whole ovine feet, tissue scrapings and biopsies taken
from the hoof using a dermatological punch. Finally, with the
knowledge of the pathology of the disease and the ability to stain
specific organisms, it was possible to perform light and electron
immuno-cytochemistry on ovine footrot lesions in order to compare
natural and experimental pathological material.

These lesions start in the interdigital space and proceed
underneath the hard horn of the hoof across the sole, around the
heel and up into the outer wall. As the lesion is propagated the
horny layers become detached from the underlying tissues and without
treatment these layers eventually slough off. Using both light and
electron microscopy the precise tissues affected by the lesion have
been studied. The lesion itself is an intraepidermal split and
passes through an area which involves the stratum granulosum and the
upper cells of the stratum spinosum. Since these layers are distal
to the germinative layer of the hoof, i.e. the stratum cylindricum,
hoof regrowth can occur if further infection does not take place.
However, exposure of the more sensitive tissues of the hoof to
bacteria such as F.necrophorum can lead to badly infected feet
which, therefore, causes considerable pain and trauma to the sheep.

Using conventional light microscopic techniques the lesion has
been shown to develop from the interdigital space which has a
structure very similar to normal skin. It then enters the soft
tissues of the hoof underlying the horn at the skin/horn junction
immediately adjacent to this area. An advanced lesion can be seen
in Figure 1 in a transverse section of one of the digits.

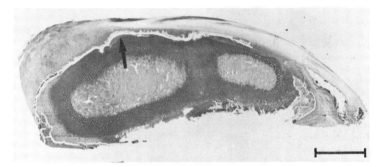

FIGURE 1: A footrot lesion (arrow) in one ovine digit. Bar = 1.0 cm

Developing lesions can show bacteria at the leading edge
(Figure 2). Apart from the fact that these bacteria are Gram
negative, the limitations of the light microscope preclude the exact
identification of these bacteria. Further information may be
obtained by use of the electron microscope.

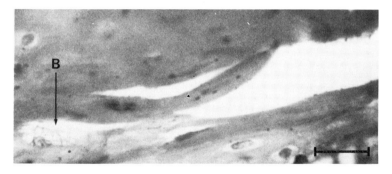

FIGURE 2: Bacteria (B) in a developing footrot lesion. Bar = 1.0 µm

Such a skin/horn junction biopsy prepared for the electron
microscope is seen in Figure 3. Here the bacteria are penetrating
under the keratinised hoof between the stratum corneum and the less
keratinised tissues. Two points should be noted. The bacteria
themselves are Gram negative rods, this being typical of hoof tissue
invasion, and this is in contrast to the large numbers of coccal
organisms seen in interdigital scrapings. Also some of the cells
are intercellular and some are intracellular, the smaller
intracellular organism has a convoluted cell wall and the
intercellular bacterium has a smooth but rather electron-lucent cell
wall structure.

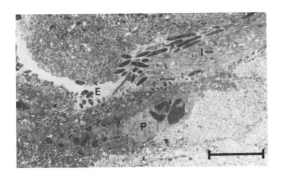

FIGURE 3:   Bacteria penetrating the skin/horn junction.
Extracellular (E) and intracellular (I) cells and a polymorphonuclear
leucocyte (P) can be seen.   Bar = 0.5 μm

Attempts have been made to demonstrate that B.nodosus produces
enzymes having the ability to attack keratin, but this situation
does not occur in vivo[7].   The role of B.nodosus as part of the
synergic infection is still poorly understood despite extensive
research into various possible determinants of virulence, such as
pili and other surface structures, elastase and protease production
(2,8,16).

The role of other bacteria in the initiation of infection has
largely been ignored.   It has been known for some time that
environmental trauma can predispose the animal to footrot and that
the establishment of the disease is dependent upon this initial
physical damage.   Recent work has shown that strains of
F.necrophorum, Bacteroides species (other than B.nodosus) and
aerobic bacilli all showing keratolytic activity can be isolated
from cases of footrot.   However, their true role remains to be
demonstrated[3,4,5].

Using electron microscopy morphological evidence for an
alternative or adjunct to the classical descriptions of the
initiation of infection can be found.

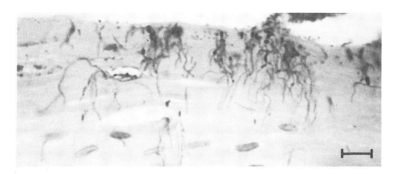

FIGURE 4: Penetration of bacteria into keratinised ovine hoof
tissue. Bar = 1.0 μm

Figure 4 shows a light micrograph of Gram negative filaments
penetrating the partially keratinised tissues. This type of
situation can be found in many cases of ovine footrot but is not
generally looked for in the hard keratinised horn where it also
often occurs. Using the light microscope there is no evidence of
natural channels or attack on the keratin matrix. However, when
seen in the electron microscope (Figure 5) bacteria are found within
the keratinised tissue. Surrounding these bacteria is an
electron-lucent space which is indicative of a keratinolytic action.

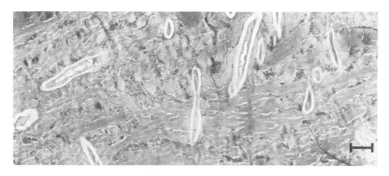

FIGURE 5: Keratinolytic bacteria penetrating the ovine hoof.
Bar = 0.1 μm

The structure of the bacteria is difficult to determine due to the nature of the tissue, but close examination sometimes reveals a thickened Gram negative cell wall which is separate from the electron-lucent space (Figure 6).

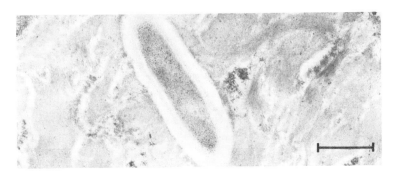

FIGURE 6: Structure of the keratolytic bacteria in footrot.
Bar = 0.05 um

The significance of this can be illustrated by returning to the ultrastructure of bacteria found in interdigital scrapings and at skin/horn junctions where a more accurate picture is obtained of the identity of the bacteria present within the developing lesion. Apart from bacteria with the morphological appearance of B.nodosus and F.necrophorum a filamentous bacterium can be found which is always in close association with F.necrophorum in the tissues. This bacterium has a Gram negative cell wall which characteristically has a low affinity for electron-dense stains. It is unusual in that it is ultrastructurally identical to the bacterium that is able to penetrate keratinised tissue directly. Upon primary isolation and subsequently under suitable conditions it is capable of forming a stable inter-bacterial relationship where a central filamentous rod is covered with a coat of smaller rods (Figure 7). Under these conditions the growth of both organisms is enhanced indicating a synergic association.

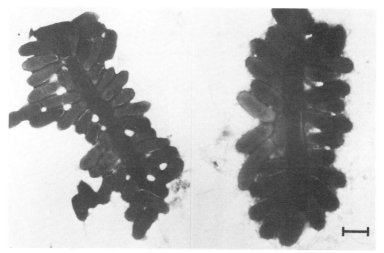

FIGURE 7: Negative stain of two 'mother and baby' configurations. Bar = 0.1 μm

Selective isolation of the two organisms allowed ultrastructural studies to be carried out. The central filament, or 'mother', has a cell wall structure similar to the filamentous bacteria found penetrating the keratinised tissues and can be shown to occur as two immunologically related colonial forms. The most stable colony variant possesses flagella but variants arise that possess no flagella but have a loose fitting capsule. The outer organisms or 'babies' have a structure similar to the convoluted wall organisms also commonly found in footrot lesions and these possess pili. In thin sections the close association of the cells may be seen to be mediated by an intercellular matrix (Figure 8).

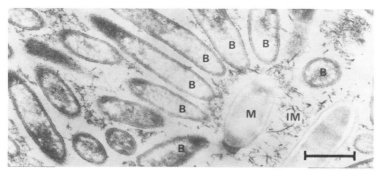

FIGURE 8: Thin section of the 'mother' (M) and 'baby' (B) configuration involving an intercellular matrix (IM). Bar = 0.05 μm

The role of this synergic association in ovine footrot requires further work for the following reasons:

1. During electron microscopic examination of natural and experimental lesions, the only organisms found consistently were those having the ultrastructure of B.nodosus, F.necrophorum and the two bacteria described here.

2. The growth characteristics and structure of the central 'mother' filament are consistent with the original descriptions of the unidentified motile fusiform of footrot[1].

3. A similar configuration commonly occurs between B.nodosus and an unidentified Gram negative rod in scrapings from footrot lesions[1,17] known as the Beveridge phenomenon (Figure 9).

4. Immunocytochemical work has shown that both these new isolates are found within footrot lesions, often in close association with F.necrophorum.

FIGURE 9: The Beveridge phenomenon in ovine footrot. Bar = 1.0 μm

Current hypotheses on the development of the footrot lesion are based upon light microscopy of tissues and correlating the morphology of the bacteria found with those isolated. To obtain definitive identification of these bacteria and also a correlation between this and the ultrastructural findings, immunocytochemical techniques were employed. All the isolates obtained from natural and experimental infection were characterized serologically and specific antisera raised against them. It was therefore possible to locate positively all isolated and characterized organisms in lesion scrapings and biopsies; by using multiple sections it was possible to relate the numbers of each isolate to one another. For example, B.nodosus was only ever found in superficial layers of lesion biopsies, either in the stratum corneum or embedded in the softer tissues where the overlying keratinised tissues had been stripped off by the passage of the lesion. F.necrophorum was always found deeper within the lesion where tissue destruction was taking place. It is interesting to note that, despite all previous reports that F.necrophorum was the only filamentous organism to be found in footrot, the newly isolated 'mother' organism was always found in close association with it. Indeed, when there were large numbers of F.necrophorum in more necrotic lesions there were correspondingly large numbers of the 'mother' organism. Thus previous ideas based on morphological evidence alone can be shown to be inadequate using this technique, and both qualitative and quantitative assessments can be made. The 'baby' organism was found to occur throughout the lesion material, but could also be found penetrating ahead of F.necrophorum in secondary infections.

CONCLUSION

(a) Current views on the pathogenicity of ovine footrot are based on four main criteria:

1. The isolation of possible causative organisms.
2. The induction of experimental disease using isolates and comparison of natural and artificial infections.
3. The investigation of infected tissue by light microscopy alone.
4. The prevention of the disease by the formulation and use of therapeutics and prophylaxis based on isolation and morphological evidence.

(b) Current research outlined here has altered these criteria by
demonstrating the following:

1. Invasion of the hoof in ovine footrot can occur in a manner
    other than the normal skin/horn junction penetration.
2. Electron microscopy can serve as a useful tool to
    investigate the role of the various tissue layers and the
    bacteria in induction and development of the lesion as it
    progresses through the hoof.
3. The structure of the bacteria present within natural and
    experimental lesions can be compared more definitively with
    that of specific bacteria isolated from infected feet.
4. Bacteria can be located specifically within the lesions
    using immunocytochemistry to complement the ultrastructural
    findings and this has also demonstrated that morphological
    similarity is not equivalent to identification.
5. Two new bacteria have been shown to occur in close
    association with the lesion as it develops, thus indicating
    that they, and possibly other bacteria, have a role in
    footrot. The fact that they are themselves synergically
    linked lends support to the synergic aspect of the disease.
6. Using the new techniques available it was possible to show
    that the experimental model using B.nodosus was similar in
    all respects to the natural infection.

(c) Future work would require the isolation and characterization of
further organisms from ovine footrot, the location of these
organisms within the lesion and an investigation of their role,
albeit active or passive. The initial stage of this has started
already with the demonstration of the two new bacteria within
active lesions and their own specific interaction.

REFERENCES

1. Beveridge WIB. (1941). Footrot in sheep: a transmissible disease due to infection with Fusiformis nodosus (n.sp). Studies on its cause, epidemiology and control. Commonwealth of Australia Council for Scientific and Industrial Research Bulletin, 140, 1-56.

2. Broad TE and Skerman TM. (1976). Partial purification and properties of extracellular proteolytic activity of Bacteroides nodosus. New Zealand Journal of Agricultural Research, 19, 317-322.

3. Cygan Z and Barcz I. (1981). Occurrence of elastolytic aerobic microflora in lameness of sheep. Medycyna weterynaryjna, 37, 284-286.

4. Cygan Z, Wiercinski J and Barcz I. (1981a). Production and specificity of proteases produced by Bacillus sp. and Corynebacterium pyogenes discovered in 'lameness' of sheep. Medycyna Weterynaryjna, 37(7), 402-404.

5. Cygan Z, Wiercinski J and Barcz I. (1981b). Gram-negative anaerobic non-sporeforming bacilli in hoof infections of sheep. Medycyna Weterynaryjna, 37(9), 513-517.

6. Egerton JR. (1979). Treatment of ovine footrot by vaccination with the specific aetiological agent Bacteroides nodosus. Comparative Immunology, Microbiology and Infectious Diseases, 2, 61-67.

7. Egerton JR, Roberts DS and Parsonson IM. (1969). The aetiology and pathogenesis of ovine footrot. I. A histological study of the bacterial invasion. Journal of Comparative Pathology, 79, 207-216.

8. Every D and Skerman TM. (1980). Ultrastructure of the Bacteroides nodosus cell envelope layers and surface. Journal of Bacteriology, 141, 845-857.

9. Katitch RV. (1979). Etiology and immunoprophylaxy problems in sheep footrot. Comparative Immunology, Microbiology and Infectious Diseases, 2, 55-59.

10. Roberts DS. (1967a). The pathogenic synergy of Fusiformis necrophorus and Corynebacterium pyogenes. I. The influence of the leucocidal exotoxin of F.necrophorus. British Journal of Experimental Pathology, 48, 665-673.

11. Roberts DS. (1967b). The pathogenic synergy of Fusiformis necrophorus and Corynebacterium pyogenes. II. The response of F.necrophorus to a filterable product of C.pyogenes. British Journal of Experimental Pathology, 48, 674-679.

12. Roberts DS. (1969). Synergic mechanisms in certain mixed infections. Journal of Infectious Diseases, 120(60), 720-724.

13. Roberts DS and Egerton JR. (1969). The aetiology and pathogenesis of ovine footrot. II. The pathogenic association of Fusiformis nodosus and F.necrophorus. Journal of Comparative Pathology, 79, 217-227.

14. Smith H. (1978). The determinants of microbial pathogenicity. In Essays in Microbiology (eds: Richmond, M.H. and Norris, J.R.), 13, 1-32. pub: Chichester J.Wiley and Sons,.

15. Smith H. (1982). The role of microbial interactions in infectious disease. Philosophical Transactions of the Royal Society of London. B. Biological Sciences, 297, 551-561.

16. Stewart DJ. (1979). The role of elastase in differentiation of Bacteroides nodosus infections in sheep and cattle. Research in Veterinary Science, 27, 99-105.

17. Sukeev Sh, Egoshin IS and Raimymbekov D. (1974). Footrot in sheep in Kirgizia: role of Fusiformis nodosus. Veterinariya, Moscow, No.3, 58-59.

A MODEL FOR INVESTIGATING POLYMORPH FUNCTION IN THE PRESENCE OF
NON-SPORING ANAEROBES

H.R. INGHAM AND PENELOPE R. SISSON

SUMMARY

At a concentration of less than 10^7 bacteria per ml,
non-sporing obligate anaerobes are phagocytosed and killed under
aerobic and anaerobic conditions, as are a range of facultative
anaerobes. At higher bacterial concentrations the phagocytic
killing of non-sporing obligate anaerobes is inhibited as is that of
concomitant faculative anaerobes; the latter do not themselves
inhibit phagocytic killing. The inhibitory effect occurs only in
the presence in the reaction mixture of suitable reducing substances
and appears to be due to an interaction between bacterial cells and
serum. Heat labile and heat stable serum factors are involved; the
interaction results in unrestricted multiplication of associated
facultative anaerobes which accumulate within polymorphs and
extracellularly.

INTRODUCTION

The possibility that obligate anaerobes might impair the action
of polymorphonuclear leucocytes (PMNL) first suggested itself to us
when observing the response to treatment, with metronidazole, of
patients with otogenic brain abscesses. These abscesses are
characterised by a mixed flora consisting of facultative and
obligate anaerobes, very reminiscent of faecal microorganisms.
Prior to the use of metronidazole as part of the chemotherapeutic
regimen for the treatment of brain abscess it was a common
experience for these patients to exhibit a slow clinical response
after aspiration of the abscess contents. This procedure had to be
repeated frequently, and the abscess contents yielded the original
microorganisms in undiminished numbers. In contrast, in patients
with otogenic brain abscess reveiving metronidazole as the

anti-anaerobic agent there was a prompt clinical response and all microorganisms disappeared rapidly. As we had varied the chemotherapy only by the substitution of metronidazole and as, at that time, this agent was thought to be without action against facultative anaerobes, it seemed possible that metronidazole might indirectly through its action on the anaerobes be removing a potentially antiphagocytic factor. We therefore established an in-vitro laboratory model to investigate this hypothesis.

MATERIALS AND METHODS

The bacterial strains and phagocytic model used in this work have been described fully elsewhere (1). Briefly, it consisted of 0.5 ml PMNL suspension in Hank's balanced salt solution (HBSS) at pH7 containing approximately 2×10^6 leucocytes/ml, 0.1 ml normal serum (on each occasion from the same patient as the phagocytes), 0.3 ml HBSS and 0.1 ml P. mirabilis (which had been grown overnight in Hartley's broth, washed thrice in physiological saline and resuspended in saline to 5×10^7 cfu/ml). Putative inhibitory organisms were grown overnight in Bacto cooked meat medium (CMM) supplemented with menadione 1 mg/L at $37^\circ C$. 0.1 ml of the resultant broth was added to the test system, and 0.1 ml of uninoculated CMM broth was added to the control tubes.

All tubes were rotated at 5 rpm aerobically or anaerobically at $37^\circ C$ for 5 h. Viable counts of P. mirabilis were performed by making ten-fold dilutions in distilled water and transferring 0.001 ml with a fused platinum-iridium loop onto MacConkey Agar. Viable counts of the anaerobic organisms were done similarly using agar containing defibrinated horse blood 5% (v/v) and nalidixic acid 50 mg/L to inhibit selectively the growth of Proteus.

RESULTS

At bacterial concentrations of less than 10^7 per ml B. fragilis was phagocytosed and killed by PMNL under aerobic and anaerobic conditions when incubated at $37^\circ C$ for 5 h. At higher concentrations, killing was inhibited as was that of P. mirabilis. This inhibitory effect was exhibited by a range of non-sporing anaerobes but not by facultative anaerobes (Tables 1 & 2).

Table 1. Effect of different inoculum levels of <u>Bacteroides fragilis</u> on phagocytic killing under aerobic conditions

Strains	Viable counts of P. mirabilis (cfu/ml)		Viable counts of B. fragilis (cfu/ml)	
	Initial	5 h	Initial	5 h
<u>Proteus mirabilis</u>	8×10^6	6×10^4		
P. mirabilis +	8×10^6	1×10^8	4×10^7	5×10^6
<u>Bacteroides fragilis</u> (U)*				
P. mirabilis +				
B. fragilis $(\frac{1}{10})$	8×10^6	1×10^5	4×10^6	1×10^3

* <u>B. fragilis</u> from an overnight culture of Bacto Cooked Meat Medium was used undiluted (U), or diluted, as shown in parenthesis, in broth from Bacto Cooked Meat Medium

The inhibitory activity of broth cultures of non-sporing anaerobes was associated with the cell fraction, there being none present in the centrifuged supernatant. High titre homologous rabbit-antiserum impaired the inhibitory activity of the cells suggesting that the effect was associated with surface components.

Inhibition of killing by PMNL was only observed in the presence of suitable reducing substances. Thus it was apparent in cultures grown in Robertsons cooked meat medium, but not in cultures in nutrient broth. The presence in the latter medium of 0.1% ascorbic acid or 1% glucose allowed, however, expression of the inhibitory effect.

Intact whole cells of <u>B. asaccharolyticus</u> at a concentration of 10^7 per ml inhibited phagocytic killing. After ultrasonic disruption no inhibition was apparent although the addition to the mixture of as few as 100 intact cells restored the activity (Table 3).

Table 2. Effect of different organisms on phagocytic killing of
Proteus mirabilis

Organisms	No. of strains	Inhibitory Index Range	Mean
ANAEROBES			
B. melaninogenicus	12	2,000-40,000	15,000
B. fragilis	13	100-20,000	6,000
B. ruminicola	3	100-500	350
Veillonella	3	200-600	333
AEROBES			
Escherichia coli	18	1-40	11
Klebsiella pneumoniae	3	1-30	10
K. atlantae	5	1-30	10
P. mirabilis	1	1	1
P. stuarti	2	1	1
Streptococcus	7	1-80	15

Table 3. Effect of ultrasonic disruption on inhibitory activity of
Bacteroides asaccharolyticus

Intact cells/ml	Inhibitory* index	Sonicated cells/ml	Inhibitory index
10^8	330	10^8	8

Intact cells/ml		Intact cells/ml	+	Sonicated cells/ml	
10^5	5	10^5		10^8	600
10^4	1	10^4		10^8	500
10^3	1	10^3		10^8	1400
10^2	10	10^2		10^8	1400

* Ratio of the viable count at 4 h of P. mirabilis in the presence
of, to that in the absence of, B. asacharolyticus.

The primary interaction appeared to be between the anaerobe and
serum. Pre-treatment of the serum with anaerobes which were then
removed by centrifugation, inhibited subsequent killing of
P. mirabilis by PMNL.

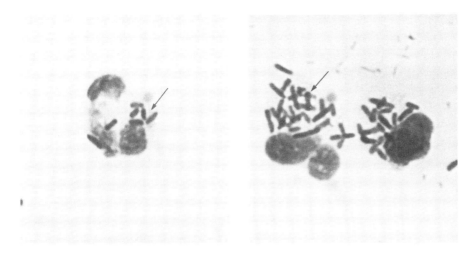

Fig. 1.   Fig. 2.

Fig. 1. Phagocytosis of a pure culture of P. mirabilis showing
polymorphonuclear leucocytes (PMNL) containing few bacteria
(arrows). Gram's stain. x 1080.

Fig. 2. Phagocytosis of a mixture of P. mirabilis and B.
asaccharolyticus showing large numbers of Proteus associated with
PMNL. Gram's stain. x 1080.

Table 4. Effect of heat-inactivation* of serum and the presence of
Bacteroides asaccharolyticus on killing of Proteum mirabilis by
phagocytes

Strain	Serum	Viable count of P. mirabilis (cfu/ml)	
		Initial	5 h
Proteus mirabilis	Normal	1×10^7	6×10^3
P. mirabilis + Bacteroides acaccharolyticus	Normal	1×10^7	3×10^6
P. mirabilis	Heat-inactivated	1×10^7	6×10^6
P. mirabilis + B. asaccharolyticus	Heat-inactivated	1×10^7	5×10^8
P. mirabilis control+		1×10^7	7×10^8

* 58°C for 20 minutes
.+ No phagocytes or serum

Killing of the latter occured when fresh, but not heat-inactivated, serum was added to the above system (Table 4). This indicated that obligate anaerobes affect the activity of a heat-labile component of serum. It seems likely that a heat-stable serum factor is also involved. Although heat inactivation impaired killing of P. mirabilis inhibition was not as marked as that seen when B. asaccharolyticus was also present.

The interaction between serum and anaerobes does not appear to interfere with engulfment of bacteria by PMNL. Gram-stained smears of the reaction mixtures at the end of incubation showed that in the presence of the anaerobe there were many organisms, large numbers of which were associated with PMNL (Figs. 1 & 2). Viable counts of the extracellular and cell-associated P. mirabilis in the presence of B. asaccharolyticus were 3×10^6 per ml and 4×10^7 respectively.

Electron microscopy of thin section of these preparations confirmed the intracellular accumulation of P. mirabilis in the presence of the anaerobe (Figs. 3 & 4). Enumeration of PMNL containing bacteria in the presence and absence of B. asaccharolyticus indicated that many more PMNL contained bacteria in the presence of the anaerobe than in its absence (Table 5). Those differences were statistically significant (P .001).

Table 5. Electron microscopic counts in thin sections of the numbers of polymorphonuclear leucocytes (PMNL) containing bacteria after incubation of Proteus mirabilis for 5 h aerobically with serum in the presence and absence of Bacteroides asaccharolyticus

Strains	Number of PMNL containing bacteria	Number of PMNL without bacteria	Total number of PMNL counted
Proteus mirabilis	59	116	175
P. mirabilis + Bacteroides asaccharolyticus	99	7	106

When PMNL were omitted from the reaction mixtures examination
of Gram-stained smears at 5 h showed that in the tubes containing
P. mirabilis and serum very few organisms were visible.   In wet
preparations however large numbers of Proteus were seen.   In the
additional presence of B. asaccharolyticus large numbers of Proteus
were seen, often in long chains and more deeply staining in
appearance.   Viable counts of P. mirabilis, however, in both
experiments were identical.

DISCUSSION

Since the inhibitory effect of non-sporing anaerobes on
phagocytic killing was first reported (2) the phenomenon has been
confirmed by other workers (3,4).   Both groups studied the
interaction between PMNL and bacteria using radioactively labelled
microorganisms, and concluded that the inhibitory effect was due to
an interaction with serum moieties which interfered with engulfment
by PMNL.   These findings, which were dependent upon observations
made during the first 45 minutes of the encounter between PMNL and
bacteria, contrast with our own observation at 5 h, when
intracellular accumulation of organisms is apparent.

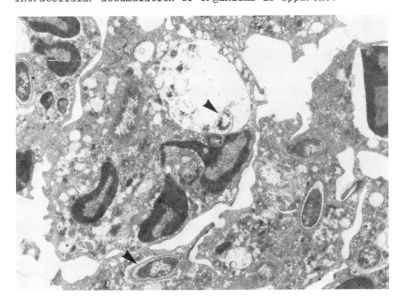

FIG 3.   Thin section of PMNL after contact with a pure culture of
         P. mirabilis showing bacteria surrounded by host-cell membrane
         (arrow) or in vacuoles in various stages of cytolysis
         (arrowheads).   EM.   x 9000.

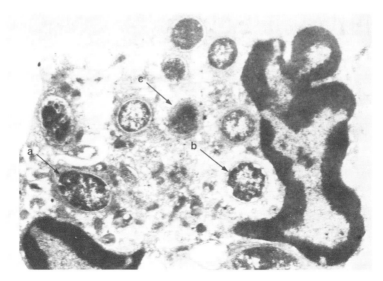

FIG. 4. Thin section of PMNL after contact with a mixture of
P. mirabilis and B. asaccharolyticus showing bacteria
surrounded by host-cell membrane (a), or in vacuoles (b), or
intracytoplasmic (c). EM. x 18,000. Electron micrographs
reproduced by courtesy of The Journal of Medical Microbiology.

These apparently conflicting observations can be reconciled if
considered in conjunction with a recent observation by Van Dyke et
al., (5) who reported that culture filtrates and cell extracts of
certain non-sporing anaerobes impair chemotaxis of PMNL.
Preliminary studies in this laboratory (unpublished data) confirm
these findings. Impairment of chemotaxis would be expected to
interfere with the engulfment of microorganisms during the early
stages of the phagocytic process, an effect entirely consistent with
the observations reported by Tofte et al., (3) and Jones and Gemmell
(4).

Our results indicate that anaerobes interfere with phagocytic
killing; engulfment appears to proceed, but subsequent killing,
inhibited. Our observations on the effect of serum on P. mirabilis,
alone, and in the presence of B. asaccharolyticus, suggest that the
anaerobe impairs the action of serum components which effect some
form of cell wall damage. This may facilitate the antibacterial
action of lysosomal contents under normal conditions. This
postulated cell wall damage, could explain the failure of serum
treated organisms to stain by the Gram technique, but is clearly not

lethal, since, in the absence of PMNL, killing of Proteus is not observed. Evidence in favour of this hypothesis can be adduced from the fact that serum-sensitive strains are no longer killed when serum is pre-treated with obligate anaerobes under the experimental conditions we have described (unpublished data).

Further studies are currently being carried out to demonstrate such serum-induced cell wall damage by methods other than susceptibility to killing by PMNL.

REFERENCES

1.   Ingham HR, Sisson PR, Tharagonnet D, Selkon JB and Codd AA. 1977. Inhibition of pharocytosis in vitro by obligate anaerobes. Lancet ii, 1252-1254.
2.   Tofte RW, Peterson PK, Schmeling D, Bracke J, Kim Y and Quie PG. 1980. Opsonization of four Bacteroides species: role of the classical complement pathway and immunoglobulin. Infect. & Immun. 27, 784-792.
3.   Jones GR and Gemmell CG. 1982. Impairment by Bacteroides species of opsonisation and phagocytosis of enterobacteria. J. Med. Microbiol. 15, 351-361.
4.   Ingham HR, Sisson PR, Middleton RL, Narang HK, Codd AA and Selkon JB. 1981. Phagocytosis and killing of bacteria in aerobic and anaerobic conditions J. Med. Microbiol. 14, 391-399.
5.   Van Dyke TE, Bartholomew E, Genco RJ, Slots J and Levine MJ. 1982. Inhibition of neutrophil chemotaxis by soluble bacterial products. J. Periodontol, 53, 502-508.

EFFECT OF BACTEROIDES FRAGILIS LIPOPOLYSACCHARIDE AND CAPSULAR POLYSACCHARIDE ON POLYMORPH FUNCTION AND SERUM KILLING

JANET C. CONNOLLY AND SOAD TABAQCHALI

1. INTRODUCTION

In clinical sepsis associated with Gram negative anaerobic rods the predominance of B. fragilis in exudate and blood suggests that it possesses some unique virulence properties. Ingham (1) has recently produced evidence of the ability of Bacteroides species to inhibit polymorph phagocytosis and killing of aerobic organisms, but the determinants responsible for this have not yet been identified. We therefore investigated the possible roles played by the lipopolysaccharide and the capsular polysaccharide of B. fragilis.

2. MATERIALS AND METHODS

Pure preparations of lipopolysaccharide and capsular polysaccharide were obtained following an extended extraction procedure originally based on that of Kasper and Seiler (2) and Kasper (3). It was found necessary to treat the capsular material twice with pronase, followed by sepharose column chromatography, in order to ensure a protein-free capsular polysaccharide preparation. Both extracts were resuspended in Hanks balanced salt solution to concentrations equivalent to those present in 10^8 whole organisms per ml (4).

An 'in vitro' phagocytosis model was set up using two strains of Proteus mirabilis as indicators of phagocytosis and killing by human polymorphs in the presence of pooled human serum. Test and control systems of constant volume were incubated at 37°C over a four hour period. Controls in each experiment included monitoring the growth of approximately 5×10^7/ml indicator organisms in Hanks balanced salt solution plus 0.1% gelatin alone, in the presence of 10% serum and with 10% serum plus 8×10^6 polymorphs/ml. The latter preparation constituted the uninhibited phagocytosis control system to which test inhibitors were added.

In some systems B. fragilis (strain ATCC 23745) was added in PYG broth to final concentrations of approximately 5×10^6/ml or 5×10^7/ml. Other tests included a combination of 5×10^6/ml B. fragilis with either purified capsular polysaccharide (at 100 ug/ml) or lipopolysaccharide (LPS) at 90 ug/ml. Capsular polysaccharide was also tested alone as an inhibitor at concentrations of 100 ug/ml or 10 ug/ml.

The potential inhibitors above were added with the indicator organisms at the start of each experiment. Viable counts of P. mirabilis were followed at Time 0 and at every hour thereafter over four hours in order to estimate killing by serum or polymorphs. Results are expressed as log increases or decreases of the indicator counts compared with those at Time 0.

Specimens were examined by light and electron microscopy at the end of the four hour incubation period and photographs were obtained. These included polymorphs in phagocytosis control systems together with low levels of B. fragilis whole cells with and without the addition of 100 ug/ml capsular material.

3.   RESULTS

Using serum-resistant strain of P. mirabilis (665)

Results are expressed as an average of three experiments. FIGURE 1 illustrates an approximate one log increase in numbers of this strain over the incubation period, growing either alone or in the presence of 10% serum. The addition of polymorphs resulted in a 0.5 log. reduction in numbers compared with those initially present (FIGURE 1).

Whole organisms of B. fragilis were added to the phagocytosis control. More than 10^7/ml inhibited phagocytosis to such a marked extent that Proteus numbers increased steadily alongside those in the growth control and those in 10% serum. Low numbers (5×10^6/ml) of Bacteroides inhibited phagocytosis to a lesser extent.

FIGURE 1

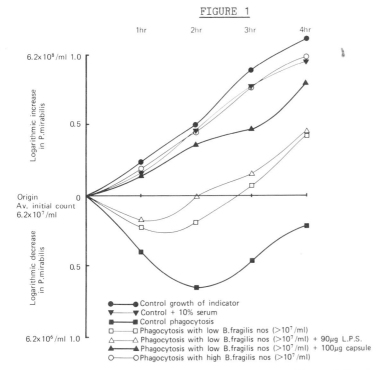

The addition of LPS to this same low concentration of B. fragilis
did not result in any further inhibition. The viable counts
obtained were similar to those obtained with B. fragilis alone as an
inhibitor. But when capsular material was added in combination with
the same levels of B. fragilis (5 x 10^6/ml), this resulted in a
marked inhibition of phagocytosis of P. mirabilis (FIGURE 1). This
was also demonstrated by the capsule alone, even at concentrations
as low as 10 ug/ml (results not shown).

Using serum-sensitive indicator strains of P. mirabilis (SBH)
Results are expressed as an average of five experiments. Numbers of
control organisms again increased steadily by approximately one log.
over the incubation period (FIGURE 2). The addition of 10% serum
demonstrated the sensitivity of the indicator strain by producing a
marked drop in the viable count over the initial two hours. After
this time, serum-lysis factors became limited and Proteus organisms
began to multiply. Polymorphs in the presence of serum produced a
similar reduction initially and it was only after the first two
hours incubation, as these curves diverged, that any further
reductions in cell numbers might be attributed to killing by
polymorphs (FIGURE 2).

The effect of whole B. fragilis organisms added to a control
phagocytosis system together with LPS or capsular material is
illustrated in Figure 3. The results of the first two hour
incubation period (Part A) were attributed as being due solely to
serum lysis. Part A demonstrates no inhibition of serum killing by
either by low levels of B. fragilis or LPS in combination with these
sub-inhibitory concentrations of B. fragilis. However, capsular
material with the same level of anaerobes reduced killing to only a
one log. reduction in cell numbers and this inhibition was yet more
marked by high levels of B. fragilis alone.

Killing by polymorphs could not be studied until the second two

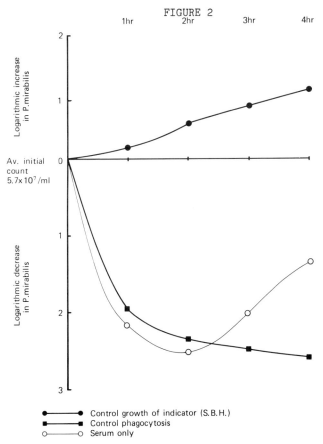

FIGURE 2

Control growth of indicator (S.B.H.)
Control phagocytosis
Serum only

hours of the experiment (Part B, FIGURE 3), when serum lysis factors
were found to be limited and the phagocytosis control graph
diverged. In part B, Proteus viable counts in inhibited test

systems tended to stabilise. There was minimal further inhibition demonstrated either by high concentrations of B. fragilis or by capsular material with low levels of the anaerobe.

Capsular polysaccharide in Hanks solution produced similar degrees of inhibition when added alone to the system at 100 ug/ml and when diluted to 10 ug/ml (FIGURE 4). The presence of whole organisms in the system therefore appeared to be unnecessary.

From these results using both a serum-sensitive and serum-resistant strain of Proteus mirabilis we postulate that B. fragilis inhibits the killing of aerobic organisms by either of two distinct mechanisms, by reducing serum lysis or by preventing phagocytic killing.

FIGURE 3

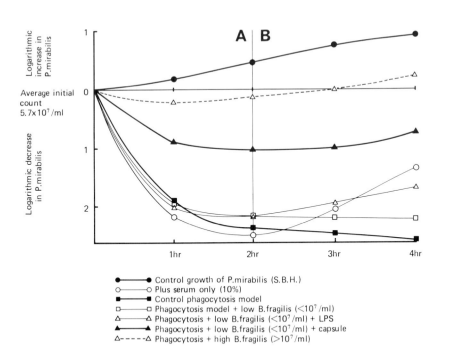

Logarithmic increase in P.mirabilis

Average initial count 5.7x10⁷/ml

Logarithmic decrease in P.mirabilis

A B

1hr   2hr   3hr   4hr

●———● Control growth of P.mirabilis (S.B.H.)
○———○ Plus serum only (10%)
■———■ Control phagocytosis model
□———□ Phagocytosis model + low B.fragilis (<10⁷/ml)
△———△ Phagocytosis + low B.fragilis (<10⁷/ml) + LPS
▲———▲ Phagocytosis + low B.fragilis (<10⁷/ml) + capsule
△-----△ Phagocytosis + high B.fragilis (>10⁷/ml)

FIGURE 4

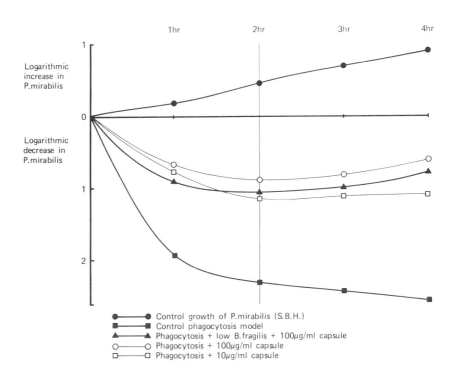

Photography. In inhibited systems, light microscopy preparations showed that the presence of B. fragilis capsular material prevented clearance of extra-cellular organisms, compared with controls. In all cases, however, polymorphs appeared to be able to engulf bacteria.

FIGURE 5 shows polymorphs containing many organisms with few bacteria remaining extracellularly. These neutrophils were photographed after four hours in a test system containing low levels of B. fragilis added to a phagocytosis control system.

FIGURE 6 demonstrates large numbers of extracellular, and non-cell associated bacteria in a system identical to that shown in FIGURE 5, except for the addition of 100 ug/ml capsular polysaccharide.

FIGURE 5

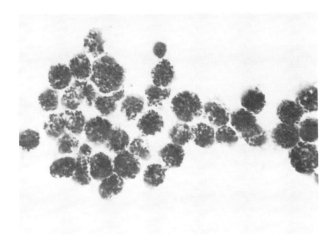

FIGURE 6

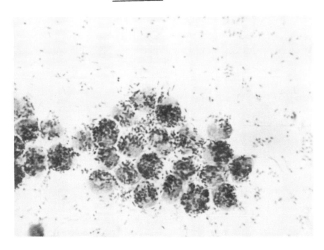

Electron micrographs indicated a reduction in degeneration of bacteria within phagosomes in inhibited systems. FIGURE 7, an EM of a polymorph from a control test, plus less than 10^7/ml B. fragilis, shows some empty vacuoles and others containing partially digested bacteria. With capsular polysaccharide added to a similar model, the polymorph appears to be unable to degrade bacteria which it has engulfed (FIGURE 8).

116

FIGURE 7

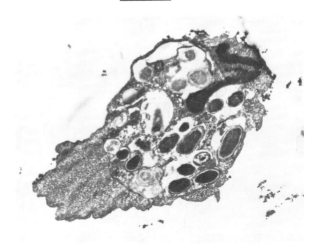

FIGURE 8

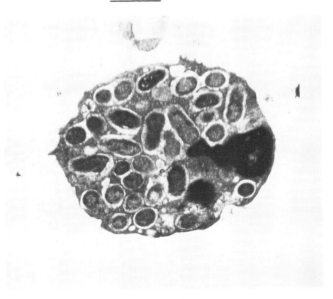

DISCUSSION

This work has indicated that the capsular polysaccharide of B. fragilis may be responsible for the inhibition of killing of aerobic organisms in an 'in-vitro' phagocytosis system. The lipopolysaccharide does not appear to have any effect.

In experiments using either indicator strain of P. mirabilis, capsular material alone at concentrations of either 100 ug/ml or 10 ug/ml inhibited killing in the absence of whole Bacteroides organisms. The presence of whole anaerobes, therefore, appears to be non-essential. Furthermore inhibition was also apparent without the inclusion of a reducing agent. This contrasts with the findings of previous workers (1) and (5) who demonstrated that inhibition of phagocytosis by anaerobes was dependent on a low redox potential in the system.

Our results indicate that inhibition of killing is mediated by a complex series of interactions. The inhibition of serum-lysis, shown by experiments using the serum-sensitive P. mirabilis indicator strain, may be due to a non-specific depletion in complement factors. Namavar et al (6) have demonstrated a heat labile component in Bacteroides gingivalis which is responsible for the inactivation of complement. Tofte et al (7) suggest from their results that competition for serum opsonins is responsible for the inhibition of killing of E. coli in a similar model.

The reduced killing by phagocytes, shown by experiments using the serum-resistant indicator, would seem to be a more specific process, as Jones and Gemmell (5) have reported that only a proportion of Proteus organisms and even fewer E. coli strains were susceptible to such inhibition by anaerobes. This may, however, be mediated by reduced opsonisation in the presence of anaerobes. It is also possible that immune complexes, activated by the anaerobic organisms, block specific receptor sites on the polymorphonuclear leucocyte membrane and thereby impair the capacity of the phagocytes to kill and degrade ingested bacteria, as shown in electron micrographs (FIGURE 8).

6. SUMMARY

Bacteroides species have recently been shown to inhibit the phagocytosis and killing of aerobic organisms. The determinants responsible for the apparent inhibition were investigated in an 'in-vitro' phagocytosis model using two strains of Proteus mirabilis as indicators. Whole organisms of B. fragilis were added as possible inhibitors of the system. Purified capsular polysaccharide and lipopolysaccharide, prepared from the same strain of B. fragilis were also tested. Results showed that more than 10^7 cfu/ml

118

Bacteroides inhibited both serum and phagocytic killing of
P. mirabilis. Concentrations below 10^7/ml had little effect on
either. Purified capsular material alone or in combination with
sub-inhibitory *B. fragilis* concentrations markedly inhibited both
serum lysis and phagocytic killing. The lipopolysaccharide appeared
to be relatively inert.

Acknowledgements

We are extremely grateful to the Wellcome Trust for funding
this project.

REFERENCES

1. Ingham HR, Sisson PR, Middleton RL. et al 1981. Phagocytosis
   and killing of bacteria in aerobic and anaerobic conditions.
   J. Med. Microbiol. 14 391-9.
2. Kasper DL and Seiler MW. 1975. Immunochemical characterization
   of the outer membrane complex of *Bacteroides fragilis*
   subspecies fragilis. J. Infect. Dis. 132 440-50.
3. Kasper DL. 1976. The polysaccharide capsule of *Bacteroides
   fragilis* subspecies fragilis: Immunochemical and morphological
   definition. J. Infect. Dis. 133 (1) 79-87.
4. Onderdonk AB, Kasper DL, Cisneros RL and Bartlett JG. 1977.
   The capsular polysaccharide of *Bacteroides fragilis* as a
   virulence factor. Comparison of the pathogenic potential of
   encapsulated and unencapsulated strains. J. Infect. Dis. 136
   82-9.
5. Jones GR and Gemmell CG. 1982. Impairment by *Bacteroides*
   species of opsonisation and phagocytosis of Enterobacteria. J.
   Med. Microbiol. 15 351-61.
6. Namavar F, Verweij Am MJJ, Bal M, et al 1983. Effect of
   anaerobic bacteria on killing of *Proteus mirabilis* by human
   polymorphonuclear leukocytes. Infection and Immunity 40 930-5.
7. Tofte RW, Peterson PK, Schmeling D, et al 1980. Opsonisation
   of four *Bacteroides* species: role of the classical complement
   pathway and immunoglobulin. Infection and Immunity 26 784-92.

THE INFLUENCE OF BACTEROIDES SP. ON THE OPSONIC ACTIVITY OF HUMAN
SERUM AND ITS EFFECT ON THE PHAGOCYTOSIS OF VARIOUS BACTERIA

C.G. GEMMELL, G.R. JONES AND R. MCNAUGHT

1. INTRODUCTION

The susceptibility of pathogenic micro-organisms to phagocytosis
by polymorphonuclear leukocytes (PMN) and macrophages is of
considerable importance in determining the outcome of the
host-parasite relationship. Pathogenic bacteria either contain or
secrete products which may interfere with this process (1). By such
means one bacterial species may interfere with the phagocytosis of
another. It has been shown that certain obligate anaerobes
including Bacteroides sp. could inhibit their own phagocytic uptake
and killing by PMN and that of other facultative anaerobes present
within their experimental system in vitro (2-5). This inhibition
depended upon a low Eh and the presence of 10^7 anaerobic
bacteria/ml (2). Interference with phagocytosis was attributed to
an impairment in the opsonic activity of the human serum used to
treat the target bacteria (3,4). When bacteroides-treated serum was
used to opsonise different Proteus species, the subsequent uptake of
all strains by PMN was inhibited, whereas the same serum inhibited
uptake of some, but not all, strains of Escherichia coli tested.
Treatment of the serum by live and dead, either heat-killed or
clindamycin-treated, bacteroides cells, elicited the same
phenomenon. In another study (5) it was recognised that the
impairment of killing of Proteus mirabilis by PMN occurred once the
bacteria were intracellular, using electron microscopy to reveal the

presence of bacteria within the phagocytic vacuoles. Others (6) have suggested that this effect is due to the production of two factors, one heat-stable and the other heat-labile, by the bacteroides cells.

In the present study we have sought to investigate more closely the interaction of the bacteroides cells with both the classical and alternative complement pathways involved in the opsonisation of different species of bacteria as a means of degining the modus operandi of the anaerobe in interfering with phagocytosis.

2. MATERIALS AND METHODS

Bacterial strains. B melaninogenicus strain no. 4 now recognised as B. asacharolyticus sub sp. melaninogenicus and Proteus mirabilis strain NGH were kindly provided by Dr. H.R. Ingham, Newcastle-upon-Tyne. The various other Bacteroides sp., Gram-positive and Gram-negative aerobic bacteria used in this study were routine isolates from the Diagnostic Bacteriology Laboratory, Glasgow Royal Infirmary.

Culture of bacteroides. All strains were grown either for 72 hours in a liquid medium consisting of cooked meat particles (Difco) reconstituted in Brain Heart Infusion Broth (Difco) to which menadione (1 ug/ml, Sigma Chemical Company, St. Louis) and haemin (5 mg/ml, Sigma) were added, or on 10% horse blood agar incubated anaerobically for 48 hours.

Radio-active labelling of cultures. All strains were cultured overnight in 20 ml of Mueller-Hinton Broth (Oxoid) containing ^{3}H-thymidine (specific activity 25Ci/mmol; Radiochemical Centre, Amersham) or ^{3}H-adenine (23Ci/mmol) at a final concentration of 10 uCi/ml broth. After incubation, the bacteria were centrifuged at 3000 g for 10 min and washed three times with 0.85% saline before use.

Opsonisation. Fresh human serum obtained from the Haematology
Department, Glasgow Royal Infirmary was stored for use in 5 ml
portions at -70°C. For opsonisation it was used at various
dilutions in Hank's balanced salt solution containing 0.1% gelatin
(gel-HBSS). The washed radio-labelled target bacterial suspensions,
standardised to contain 5×10^7 organisms/ml, were mixed with the
serum and incubated at 37°C for 15 mins with shaking and then
centrifuged at 3000 g for 10 mins. The bacterial pellet was
resuspended in gel-HBSS to its original volume.

Leucocyte preparation. Venous blood was collected from healthy
donors and heparinised (IOU heparin/ml blood). A suspension of
purified PMN was separated by dextran sedimentation and standardised
to contain 5×10^6 cells per ml HBSS (7).

Phagocytic uptake of radio-labelled bacteria by PMN followed the
method described earlier (4,8).

Measurement of complement components. Levels of C_1q and C_3
in the serum preparations used to opsonise the bacteria were
measured by radial immune haemolysis on commercially prepared plates
(Kallestad Laboratories, Austin, Texas).

Bacteroides treatment of serum. Fresh serum samples were mixed
with an equal volume of bacteroides cells (1×10^7/ml) and
incubated with shaking for up to 60 mins at 37°C. The bacteria
were removed by centrifugation at 3000 g for 10 mins and the
residual serum used to opsonise the target bacteria for use in the
phagocytosis assay.

3. RESULTS

Based upon our earlier studies (4) in which it was recognised that the efficacy of phagocytic uptake of P. mirabilis was dependent upon efficient serum opsonisation via activation of the classical complement pathway. Initial experiments showed that bacteroides treatment of serum for varying periods of time reduced the opsonic activity of that serum (table 1). In addition, the percentage serum used in these circumstances modified the inhibitory effect of the bacteroides cells on phagocytosis (table 2). It is evident that human serum even at 20% v/v gel-HBSS allowed 60% uptake of P. mirabilis within 15 mins whereas, under the same conditions, serum pretreated with either B. fragilis or B. melaninogenicus only allowed the uptake of 10.6 and 3.1% respectively of the target bacteria by the PMN.

Table 1. Effect of serum interaction time with bacteroides cells on opsonic activity for P. mirabilis

Serum contact time (mins)	% uptake of P. mirabilis by human PMN*
0	62 $\pm$ 4
15	12 $\pm$ 2
30	3 $\pm$ 2
60	2 $\pm$ 2

* expressed on the mean of three experiments with different preparations of PMN

Table 2. Effect of serum concentration on opsonization of
         P. mirabilis by bacteroides-treated serum

	*Percentage uptake of P. mirabilis after opsonization in			
Serum opsonin	50% Serum	25% Serum	20% Serum	10% Serum
Normal serum	81.7	66.4	60.7	23.2
B.fragilis-treated serum	47.5	13.7	10.6	0.0
B.melaninogenicus-treated serum	38.2	5.4	3.1	1.9

* mean of at least three experiments

When the levels of C_1q and C_3 were measured in serum samples
following their incubation with P. mirabilis alone or after
pretreatment with B. melaninogenicus or B. fragilis (table 3) it was
apparent that the presence of bacteroides cells did not reduce the
amounts of C_1q and C_3 in the serum, compared to that found in
their absence. This suggests that activation of the classical
complement cascade is impaired by the bacteroides cells such that
the normal opsonisation of P. mirabilis, via this pathway, did not
take place.

Table 3. Effect of Bacteroides sp. on two serum complement
         components with respect to opsonisation of P. mirabilis

	Effect on levels of	
Serum Treatment	C_1q	C_3
P. mirabilis	reduced	reduced
B.melaninogenicus	none	none
as above + P.mirabilis	Little effect	Little effect
B.fragilis	none	none
as above + P.mirabilis	Little effect	Little effect

The opsonisation and subsequent phagocytosis of bacteria other than P. mirabilis was examined in a similar way following serum pretreatment with bacteroides cells. With a variety of Gram-positive and Gram-negative bacteria it became apparent that impairment of opsonisation occurred quite generally among Gram-negative aerobic organisms, but not among Gram positive bacteria such as staphylococci and Streptococcus faecalis (table 4). In only two strains of staphylococcus (both were coagulase-negative) and in no strain of S. faecalis was opsonization affected by bacteroides pretreatment of the serum.

Table 4.   Survey of bacterial strains with respect to serum opsonin
            impairment by B.melaninogenicus

Organism	Strains tested	No. of strains showing opsonic inhibition by B.melaninogenicus
Proteus sp.	10	10/10
E. coli	11	7/11
Klebsiella sp.	10	7/10
Enterobacter sp.	10	6/10
Pseudomonas sp.	9	7/9
S. faecalis	9	0/9

Some impairment of opsonization of S. aureus however could be demonstrated either when the opsonising serum was pretreated with bacteroides cells for a longer period of time (up to 60 min) or when lower serum concentrations were used. Usually S. aureus can be adequately opsonised with 10% human serum but some impairment by bacteroides cells was seen after 30 or 60 min rather than 15 min as hitherto used for P. mirabilis (see Fig 1). It should also be noted that B. fragilis whose serum opsonisation is fairly resistant to impairment by another bacteroides cell over 15 mins is impaired by 60 min pretreatment. This is likely to be due to straight competition for the same opsonins via the alternative complement pathway.

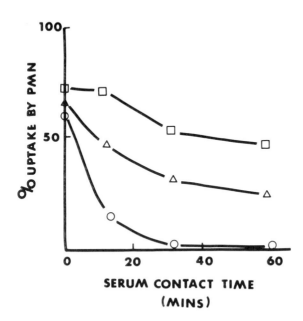

Figure 1   Effect of bacteroides-serum contact time on opsonisation
           and subsequent uptake of S. aureus, B. fragilis and
           P. mirabilis by PMN.

                        S. aureus opsonised in 10% serum
                        B. fragilis opsonised in 20% serum
                        P. mirabilis opsonised in 20% serum

Lowering the serum content of the opsonic source to 2.5% increased
the degree of impairment of opsonisation induced by bacteroides (Fig
2). Only 40% of the target staphylococci were ingested by the PMN
following bacteroides treatment of the serum compared to 74% in the
absence of the anaerobe.

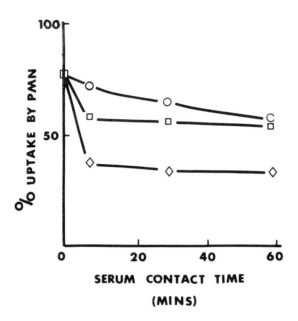

Figure 2   Effect of bacteroides-serum contact time on opsonisation
and subsequent uptake of S. aureus by PMN.

S. aureus opsonised in 10% serum
S. aureus opsonised in 5% serum
S. aureus opsonised in 2.5% serum

4.   DISCUSSION

These results confirm and extend earlier findings (2,4) and
place the phenomenon of bacterial interference with phagocytosis on
a firmer biological basis. The theory (3) that competition for
serum opsonins was critical in this respect, has been amplified in
the present study using different target bacteria and varying
opsonic conditions. It appears that the bacteroides cells owe their
activity, not to the impairment of the alternative complement
pathway utilized by most Gram-positive bacteria, but to an action on
the classical pathway utilized by most Gram-negative bacteria. Our
measurements of complement levels in each experimental system would
support this concept. Earlier studies (4) had shown that inhibition
of the classical pathway by ethyleneglycol-bis-(B-aminoethyl-ether)
N,N'-tetra-acetic acid (EGTA) failed to affect the opsonic
impairment by bacteroides cells.

We have shown an important difference between Gram-positive and Gram-negative bacteria in terms of the interference caused to their uptake, by PMN by bacteroides cells. The Gram-positive bacteria under normal circumstances were less susceptiblel to opsonic interference as well as exhibiting a lower killing index (2). Manipulation of the opsonic conditions however (serum concentration and contact time) could reverse the comparative immunity of this strain of Staphylococcus aureus.

Previous studies have shown that the killing of P. mirabilis by PMN was affected by the anaerobe - serum interaction (5,6). Both groups showed that intracellular killing measured by light and electron microscopy and by chemiluminescence were impaired in the presence of bacteroides cells. In addition, Namavar et al (6) suggested that a heat-labile and a heat-stable extracellular factor are involved in this phenomenon. The heat labile component interacted with the complement system while the heat-stable component could modify PMN killing of P. mirabilis without directly damaging the PMN.

There is now strong experimental evidence that the clinical association of large numbers of anaerobic bacteria and facultatively anaerobic enteric bacteria in intra-abdominal sepsis (9) might, in part, be explained by impairment of the phagocytosis by the anaerobe. Further studies are necessary to determine whether similar findings occur in vivo. Reznikow et al. (10) showed that the clearance of E.coli from the peritoneal cavity of mice occurred at the same rate whether or not B.fragilis was also injected into the animals. However, it is unlikely that this model mirrors adequately the serum - bacterium - phagocyte interaction demonstrable in vitro; a skin abscess might be a more appropriate system to study.

128

REFERENCES

1. Quie PG, Giebink GS, Peterson PK. 1981. Bacterial mechanisms
    for inhibition of ingestion by phagocytic cells. In Microbial
    perturbation of host defences edited by F O'Grady and H Smith,
    London Academic Press, p.121-141.
2. Ingham HR, Sisson PR, Tharagonnet D, Selkon JB, Codd AA. 1977.
    Inhibition of phagocytosis in vitro by obligate anaerobes.
    Lancet 2, 1252-1254.
3. Tofte RW, Peterson PK, Schmeling D, Bracke J, Kim Y, Quie PG.
    1980. Opsonization of four Bacteroides sp.: role of the
    classical complement pathway and immunoglobulin. Infection and
    Immunity 26, 784-792.
4. Jones GR, Gemmell CG. 1982. Impairment by Bacteroides species
    of opsonisation and phagocytosis of enterobacteria. J. Med.
    Microbiol. 15, 351-361.
5. Ingham HR, Sisson PR, Middleton RL, Narang HK, Codd AA, Selkon
    JB. 1981. Phagocytosis and killing of bacteria in aerobic and
    anaerobic conditions. J. Med. Microbiol. 14, 391-399.
6. Namavar F, Vermeij AMJJ, Bal M, van Steenbergen TJM, de Graaf
    J, MacLaren DM. 1983. Effect of anaerobic bacteria on killing
    of Proteus mirabilis by human polymorphonuclear leukocytes.
    Infection and Immunity 40, 930-935.
7. Boyum A. 1968. Separation of leukocytes from blood and bone
    marrow. Scand. J. Clin. Lab. Invest. 21, (Suppl.97), 77-89.
8. Verhoef J, Peterson PK, Quie PG. 1977. Kinetics of
    staphylococcal opsonisation, attachment, ingestion and killing
    by human polymorphonuclear leukocytes: a quantitative assay
    using (^{3}H)-thymidine-labelled bacteria. J. Immunol. Methods
    14, 303-311.
9. Joiner KA, Gelfand JA, Onderdonk AB, Bartlett JG, Gorbach SL.
    1980. Host factors in the formation of abscesses. J. Infect.
    Dis. 142, 40-49.
10. Reznikov M, Finlay-Jones JJ, McDonald PJ. 1981. Effect of
    Bacteroides fragilis on the peritoneal clearance of Escherichia
    coli in mice. Infection and Immunity 32, 398-399.

IN VITRO AND IN VIVO STUDIES ON THE PERTUBATION OF HOST DEFENCE BY
BLACK-PIGMENTED BACTEROIDES SPECIES.

G. SUNDQVIST AND J. CARLSSON

The black-pigmented Bacteroides sp. have for a long time
attracted the attention of bacteriologists because of their
suspected role in the pathogenesis of polymicrobial infections. All
anaerobic rods producing black-pigmented colonies when grown on
blood agar were initially classified as one species, Bacterium
melaninogenicum (1). Later, the name Bacteroides melaninogenicus
was established (2). This species was subsequently divided by
Holdeman and Moore (3) into three subspecies, melaninogenicus,
intermedius, and asaccharolyticus. These subspecies proved,
however, to be heterogeneous, and the following new species were
created: B. melaninogenicus, B. loescheii and B. denticola from
subspecies melaninogenicus (4); B. intermedius and B. corporis from
subspecies intermedius (5); and B. asaccharolyticus and B.
gingivalis from subspecies asaccharolyticus (6). This new
classification has been of great help in recent studies on the
pathogenic potential of these bacteria.

B. gingivalis and B. intermedius are the most common species of
black-pigmented Bacteroides in the oral cavity. They are
principally found in gingival pockets in association with different
forms of periodontal disease, but they are also often isolated from
other purulent infections in the jaws (7,8). B. melaninogenicus is
isolated, in low frequency from the oral cavity or from clinical
infections (7,9,10). B. asaccharolyticus colonizes the human

intestinal tract and is isolated from clinical infections (9), but is not found in the oral cavity (6,11). The original information about the pathogenicity of the black-pigmented Bacteroides sp. came from studies on the infectious potential of the indigenous human microbiota. In experimental animals inoculated subcutaneously with dental scrapings, or with human faecal suspensions, necrotic infections developed. In these infections, which were polymicrobial, black-pigmented Bacteroides sp. were regularly recovered (12-15). Elucidation of the specific role of the individual bacteria revealed that black-pigmented Bacteroides sp. were indispensible for the development of the infections (14-15). At the time of these studies the various black-pigmented Bacteroides sp. had not been classified, but Macdonald et al. (14) showed that both saccharolytic and asaccharolytic strains could participate in the infections, while Mayrand et al. (16) later reported that only B. gingivalis, in combination with a mixture of five non-characterised bacterial strains, was infective. The ability of this combination to induce infections was lost when B. gingivalis was substituted with saccharolytic black-pigmented Bacteroides strains. Recent studies have, however, shown that B. intermedius can also be a key organism in inducing polymicrobial infections (17,18).

The infections that developed in the animals inoculated with the indigenous microbiota were of two types (14,15), either localized purulent abscesses or spreading necrotic lesions, usually accompanied by bacteraemia. In a later study the spreading necrotic infections were associated with the presence of B. gingivalis in the infective mixtures (16). Black-pigmented Bacteroides sp. may also, however, induce infections in pure culture. Burdon (19) reported that one strain, in pure culture, inoculated subcutaneously in guinea pigs, produced an extensive cutaneous gangrene with death of the animals in about 48 hours. Strains pathogenic in pure culture in guinea pigs or rabbits, have also been reported (14,18,20-23). In recent studies, concentrated fresh bacterial suspensions were inoculated subcutaneously and the tissue reactions were examined

microscopically, giving important information about the virulence of
the various black-pigmented species (22,23). Strains of
B. gingivalis produced rapidly spreading infections, which resulted
in either gravity or phlegmonous abscesses and frequently killed the
animals. B. intermedius caused localized abscesses. There were,
however, some variation in pathogenicity among the strains within
these two species; strains of B. melaninogenicus and
B. asaccharolyticus were, usually, much less virulent than strains
of the other two species.

Early observations on the virulence factors of the
black-pigmented Bacteroides sp. showed that they could be
proteolytic (19), act on blood substances (24) and produce
fibrinolysin (25). Among an array of lytic enzymes produced by
these bacteria (7) the collagenolytic activity (26) has attracted
most of the attention. Strains with high collagenolytic activity
were more infective than strains with weak activity (16, 27). It
was also shown that a cell-free extract of a B. gingivalis strain
with collagenolytic activity enhanced a fusobacterial infection and
gave a more severe abscess formation than either the extract or the
fusobacterial strain alone (28).

Lipopolysaccharides are important virulence factors of many
facultatively anaerobic Gram-negative bacteria. The
lipopolysaccharides of the black-pigmented Bacteroides are, however,
chemically distinct from the lipopolysaccharides of the
facultatively anaerobic Gran-negative bacteria (29) in that they
lack two core sugars (2-keto-3-deoxyoctonate and heptose) as well as
B-hydroxymyristic acid (the predominant fatty acid in the lipid A
moiety). They have low endotoxic activity (30,31) and do not seem
to play any major role in the pathogenicity of the organisms.

The virulence of many strains of black-pigmented Bacteroides sp.
is dependent on the other bacteria present in the infective mixtures
(14,16,18) but, although these other bacteria may be indispensable

in these infections, they do not possess any abvious virulence
factors. Their major role seem to be to provide the black-pigmented
Bacteroides sp. with growth factors such as vitamin K, haemin or
succinate (14,32-34).

An important observation, in the experimental infections, was
that the black-pigmented Bacteroides sp. survived in the abscesses
despite a massive migration of polymorphonuclear leucocytes into the
site of infection. The ability to resist phagocytosis, or
intracellular killing was one important way in which the
black-pigmented Bacteroides sp. perturbed the host defence (18). It
has been reported that a highly virulent saccharolytic strain of
black-pigmented Bacteroides, which had a capsule, was not readily
phagocytosed and killed in an in vitro system (35) and that
encapsulated strains induced experimental polymicrobial abscesses in
contrast to non-encapsulated strains (36). Another important
observation from these experimental infections was that the bacteria
inoculated together with the black-pigmented Bacteroides sp. also
survived in the tissues (18). This suggested that the
polymorphonuclear leucocytes at the site of infection had an
impaired function.

It has been shown in vitro that the black-pigmented Bacteroides
sp. inhibited, not only their own serum-dependent phagocytosis
and/or killing, but also that of other bacteria (37-41). Ingham et
al (37,38) concluded from their studies that black-pigmented
Bacteroides sp. affected serum in such a way that it allowed the
engulfment of the organisms by the leucocytes but markedly impaired
their intracellular killing. The conclusion of Tofte et al (39) and
of Jones and Gemmell (40) was that there was competition between
black-pigmented Bacteroides sp. and other bacteria, for serum
opsonins and this reduced the capacity of the leucocytes to
phagocytose. Namavar et al (41) found a leukocyte inhibitory factor
in the culture filtrate of B. gingivalis, which was heat-stable and
had a molecular weight of less than 3500.

The interaction between phagocytes and black-pigmented
Bacteroides sp. has also been studied with the chemiluminescence
assay. Leucocytes increase their oxidative metabolism during
phagocytosis and emit light (chemiluminescence) as a result of this
metabolic activity (42,43). Considerable differences were found
among the various black-pigmented Bacteroides sp. in their ability
to induce chemiluminescence. Strains of B. intermedius,
B. melaninogenicus, and B. loescheii were much more efficient in
activating the leucocytes than strains of B. gingivalis. Among
strains of B. gingivalis, the most virulent strains had much less
capacity to activate the leukocytes than the other strains (42).

The complement system and antibodies play an important role in
the battle of the polymorphonuclear leucocytes against infections
caused by pyogenic microogranisms. The complement components are
the source of chemotactic peptides and heat-labile opsonins, which
facilitate recognition and killing of the microorganisms by the
leucocytes. The antibodies participate in the activation of the
complement, and also work as opsonins. If these vital functions are
jeopardized, the host defence against infections is dangerously
compromised.

Kilian (44) showed that IgA, IgG and IgM were degraded by
strains of B. asaccharolyticus, B. gingivalis and B. intermedius,
but not by strains of B. melaninogenicus. A strain of
B. asaccharolyticus degrades not only the immunoglobulins, but also
a wide array of other human plasma proteins (45). With this ability
to degrade immunoglobulins, the black-pigmented Bacteroides sp.
obviously have the capacity to paralyse significant parts of the
host defence against infections.

In a recent study B. gingivalis and B. intermediums were
inoculated into subcutaneously implanted tissue cages in guinea pigs
(46), making it possible to study the humoral and cellular responses

against these infections. Although the numbers of polymorphonuclear leucocytes that accumulated in the tissue cages as a response to the various strains were similar, the tissue response around the cages varied with the strains, and was also influenced by the size of the infective dose. Localized abscesses were induced by strains of B. intermedius, while B. gingivalis caused a spreading, purulent breakdown of the tissue and death of the animals. The high pathogenicity of B. gingivalis could be correlated with a high proteolytic activity and degradation of immunoglobulins and the C3 protein of complement at the site of infection. The high proteolytic activity of B. gingivalis against plasma was confirmed in vitro by incubating B. gingivalis with guinea-pig serum. With 10^9 organisms added to 1 ml of serum and incubated at $37^{\circ}C$, not only the C3 protein and the immunoglobulins, but also most other serum proteins, were completely degraded within 24 h. This characteristic of B. gingivalis would certainly be of great importance in its perturbation of the host defence, and would explain the spreading of the infection in the tissues.

The key role of the plasma opsonins in the host defence was illustrated by the finding that two strains (W83 and 381) of B. gingivalis were similarly effective in degrading the C3 protein of complement, immunoglobulins, and other plasma proteins, but serum was only required to activate the leucocytes against one (W83) of the strains (42) and only that strain was highly virulent. The most plausible explanation for its pathogenicity was that by degrading the plasma opsonins, it efficiently perturbed the leucocytic host defence. Serum was not required to activate the leukocytes against strain 381 (42) and that strain was non-virulent. The ability of that strain to degrade plasma proteins probably did not hamper the host defence because the leucocytes could phagocytose and kill it, irrespective of the presence of plasma opsonins. The capacity to degrade the plasma opsonins thus appeared to be the most important virulence factor of B. gingivalis strain W83. The virulence factors of other black-pigmented Bacteroides strains remain to be demonstrated.

REFERENCES

1. Oliver WW, and Wherry WB. 1921. Notes on some bacterial
    parasites of the human mucous membranes. J. Infect. Dis.
    28:341-345.
2. Roy TE, and Kelly CD. 1939. Genus VIII Bacteroides Castellani
    and Chalmers, p. 556-558. In: Bergey's Manual of
    Determinative Bacteriology (Bergey DH, Breed RS, Murray EGD and
    Hitchens AP. ed.), 5th edn. Baltimore: The Williams and
    Wilkins Co.
3. Holdeman LV and Morre WEC. 1974. Genus I. Bacteroides
    Castellani and Chalmers 1919. p. 385-404. In: Bergey's
    Manual of Determinative Bacteriology (Buchanan RE and Gibbons
    NE. ed.), 8th edn. Baltimore: The William and Wilkins Co.
4. Holdeman LV and Johnson JL. 1982. Description of _Bacteroides_
    loescheii sp. nov. and emendation of the descriptions of
    Bacteroides melaninogenicus (Oliver and Wherry) Roy and Kelly
    1939 and _Bacteroides denticola_ Shah and Collins 1981. Int. J.
    Syst. Bacteriol. _32_:399-409.
5. Johnson JL and Holdeman LV. 1983. _Bacteroides intermedius_
    comb. nov. and descriptions of _Bacteroides corporis_ sp. nov.
    and _Bacteroides levii_ sp. nov. Int. J. Syst. Bacteriol.
    _33_:15-25.
6. Coykendall AL, Kaczmarek FS and Slots J. 1980. Genetic
    heterogeneity in _Bacteroides asaccharolyticus_ (Holdeman and
    Moore 1970) Finegold and Barnes 1977 (Approved Lists, 1980) and
    proposal of _Bacteroides gingivalis_ sp. nov. and _Bacteroides_
    macacae (Slots and Genco) comb. nov. Int. J. Syst. Bact.
    _30_:559-564.
7. Slots J. 1982. Importance of black-pigmented Bacteroides in
    human periodontal disease, p. 27-45. In: Host-parasite
    interactions in periodontal diseases (Genco RJ and Mergenhagen
    SE. ed.). Washington D.C.: American Society for Micribiology.
8. Bartlett JG and O'Keefe P. 1979. The bacteriology of
    perimandibular space infections. J. Oral Surg. 37:407-409.
9. Holdeman LV, Cato EP and Moore WEC. 1974. Current
    clasification of clinically important anaerobes, p.67-78. In:
    Anaerobic bacteria: Role in disease (Balows A, DeHaan RM,
    Dowell VR and Guze LB, ed.). Springfield: Charles C. Thomas.
10. Spiegel CA, Hayduk SE, Minah GE and Krywolap GN. 1979.
    Black-pigmented Bacteroides from clinically characterized
    peridontal sites. J. Peridont. Res. _14_:376-382.
11. Slots J and Genco RJ. 1979. Direct hemagglutination technique
    for differentiating _Bacteroides asaccharolyticus_ oral strains
    from nonoral strains. J. Clin. Microbiol. _10_:371-373.
12. Hite KE, Locke M and Hesseltine HC. 1949. Synergism in
    experimental infection with nonsporulating anaerobic bacteria.
    J. infect. Dis. _84_:1-9.

13. MacDonald JB, Sutton RM, Knoll ML, Madlener EM and Grainger RM. 1956. The pathogenic components of an experimental fusospirochetal infection. J. Infect. Dis. 98:15-20.

14. MacDonald JB, Socransky SS and Gibbons RJ. 1963. Aspects of the pathogenesis of mixed anaerobic infections of mucous membranes. J. Dent. Res. 42:529-544.

15. Socransky SS and Gibbons RJ. 1965. Required role of Bacteroides melaninogenicus in mixed anaerobic infections. J. Infect. Dis. 113:247-253.

16. Mayrand D, McBride BC, Edwards T and Jensen S. 1980. Characterization of Bacteroides asaccharolyticus and B. melaninogenicus oral isolates. Can. J. Microbiol. 26:1178-1183.

17. Sundqvist GK. 1976. Bacteriological studies of necrotic dental pulps. Odontological dissertation No. 7. University of Umea, Sweden.

18. Sundqvist GK, Eckerbom MI, Larsson AP and Sjogren UT. 1979. Capacity of anaerobic bacteria from necrotic dental pulps to induce purulent infections. Infect. Immun. 25:685-693.

19. Burdon KL. 1932. Isolation and cultivation of Bacterium melaninogenicum. Proc. Soc. Exp. Biol. 29:1144-1145.

20. Pulverer G and Heinrich S. 1960. Infektionsversuche an Laboratioriumstieren und in vitro-Untersuchungen zur Fermentausstattung des Bacteroides-melaninogenicus. Z. Hyg. 146:341-349.

21. Takazoe I, Tanaka M and Homma T. 1971. A pathogenic strain of Bacteroides melaninogenicus. Arch. Oral Biol. 16:817-822.

22. Kastelein P, van Steenbergen TJM, Bras JM and de Graaff J. 1981. An experimentally induced phelgmonous abscess by a strain of Bacteroides gingivalis in guinea pigs and mice. Antonie van Leeuwenhoek 47:1-9.

23. Van Steenbergen TJM, Kastelein P, Touw JJA, de Graaff J. 1982. Virulence of black-pigmented Bacteroides strains from periodontal pockets and other sites in experimentally induced skin lesions in mice. J. Peridontal Res. 17:41-49.

24. Shevkey M, Kohl C and Marshall MS. 1934. Bacterium melaninogenicum. J. Lab. Clin. Med. 19:689-694.

25. Weiss C. 1937. Observations on Bacterium melaninogenicum: demonstration of fibrinolysin, pathogenicity and serological types. Proc. Soc. Exp. Biol. 37:437-476.

26. Gibbons RJ and MacDonald JB. 1961. Degradation of collagenous substrates by Bacteroides melaninogenicus. J. Bacteriol. 81:614-621.

27. Kestenbaum RC, Massing J and Weiss S. 1964. The role of collagenase in mixed infections containing Bacteroides melaninogenicus. J. Dent. Res., Suppl., 43:747-748.

28. Kaufman EJ, Mashimo PA, Hausmann E, Hanks CT and Ellison SA. 1972. Fusobacterial infection: enhancement by cell-free extracts of Bacteroides melaninogenicus possessing collagenolytic activity. Arch. Oral Biol. 17:577-580.
29. Mansheim BJ, Onderdonk AB and Kasper DL. 1978. Immunochemical and biologic studies of the lipopolysaccharide of Bacteroides melaninogenicus subspecies asaccharolyticus. J. Immunol. 120:72-78.
30. Hofstad T. 1969. Serological properties of lipopolysaccharide from oral strains of Bacteroides melaninogenicus. J. Bacteriol. 97.:1078-1082.
31. Sveen K. 1977. The capacity of lipopolysaccharides from Bacteriodes, Fusobacterium and Veillonella to produce skin inflammation and the local and generalized Schwartzman reaction in rabbits. J. Periodont. Res. 12:340-350.
32. Lev M. 1958. Apparent requirement for vitamin K of rumen strain of Fusiformis nigrescens. Nature 87:203.
33. Lev M, Keudell KC and Milford AF. 1971. Succinate as a growth factor for Bacteroides melaninogenicus. J. Bacteriol. 108:175-178.
34. Mayrand D. and McBride BC. 1980. Ecological relationships of bacteria involved in a simple mixed anaerobic infection. Infect. Immun. 27:44-50.
35. Okuda K and Takazoe I. 1973. Antiphagocytic effects of the capsular structure of a pathogenic strain of Bacteroides melaninogenicus. Bull. Tokyo Dent. Coll. 14:99-104.
36. Takazoe I, Okuda K and Yamamoto A. 1975. Distribution of a K-antigen among oral strains of Bacteroides melaninogenicus. Bull. Tokyo Dent. Coll. 16:1-5.
37. Ingham H.R, Sisson PR, Tharagonnet D, Selkon JB and Codd AA. 1977. Inhibition of pharocytosis in vitro by obligate anaerobes. Lancet 2:1252-1254.
38. Ingham HR, Sisson PR, Middleton RL, Narang HK, Codd AA and Selkon JB. 1981. Phagocytosis and killing of bacteria in aerobic and anaerobic conditions. J. Med. Microbiol. 14:391-399.
39. Tofte RW, Peterson PK, Schmeling D, Bracke J, Kim Y. and Quie PG. 1980. Opsonization of four Bacteroides species: Role of the classical complement pathway and immunoglobulins. Infect. Immun. 27:784-792.
40. Jones GR and Gemmell CG. 1982. Impairment by Bacteroides species of opsonisation and phagocytosis of enterobacteria. J. Med. Microbiol. 15:351-361.
41. Namaver F, Vermeij AMJJ, Bal M, van Steenbergen TJM, de Graaff J, and MacLaren DM. 1983. Effect of anaerobic bacteria on killing of Proteum mirabilis by human polymorphonuclear leukocytes. Infect. Immun. 40:930-935.
42. Van Steenbergen TJM. 1981. Classification and virulence of black-pigmented Bacteroides strains. Dissertation. Vrije Universiteit Amsterdam The Netherlands.

138

43. Sundqvist G., Bloom GD, Enberg K and Johansson E. 1982. Phagocytosis of Bacteroides melaninogenicus and Bacteroides gingivalis in vitro by human neutrophils. J. Peridont. Res. 17:113-121.

44. Kilian M. 1981. Degradation of immunoglobulins A1, A2, and G by suspected principal peridontal pathogens. Infect. Immun. 34:757-765.

45. Werner H and Muller HE. 1971. Immunoelektrophoretische Untersuchungen uber die Einwirkung von Bacteroides-, Fusobacterium-, Leptotrichia- und Spaerophorus-Arten auf menschliche Plasmaproteine. Zbl Bakt I. Abt. Orig. 216:96-113.

46. Sundqvist GK, Carlsson J, Hermann BF, Hofling JF and Vaatainen A. 1984. Degradation in vivo of the C3 protein of guinea-pig complement by a pathogenic strain of Bacteroides gingivalis. Scand. J. Dent. Res. In press.

IN VITRO METABOLISM IN THE RUMEN FERMENTATION

R.E. HUNGATE

SUMMARY

The effects of gut microbes on many aspects of host biology can be studied by removing the gut contents and determining the effect of selected treatments on their activity in vitro. Results of these studies are complementary to those obtained with axenic microbes and animals, and in many instances can be obtained more easily and be more pertinent than results of studies on pure cultures. The zero time rate method for studying a natural microbial ecosystem is described, and a number of examples of its application to the rumen are presented.

INTRODUCTION

Gut contents are a part of the environment external to the animal even though sequestered within it. The temperature, moisture, food, and absence of molecular oxygen make this environment extremely favorable for continuous microbial growth. A teeming population of myriads of individuals composing hundreds of species of bacteria and protozoa has developed, constituting a gut environment completely different from that to which the external surfaces of the animal are exposed.

The importance of the gut ecosystem makes its quantitative description desirable. Several questions can indicate the information needed for the description: (a) Can the ecosystem be defined in space and its abiotic features such as temperature, moisture, solutes and substrates be described? (b) What organisms occupy the ecosystem? This involves isolation of each biotic component, including the animal, in axenic (pure) culture. (c) What do they do and how much? This includes identification and measurement of rates of activities in pure cultures. These activities are not necessarily the same as those performed in the ecosystem; their pertinence to the rumen must be confirmed. (d) What does the total ecosystem do and how much? This can be accomplished by removing the gut ecosystem and measuring its rates of activity _in vitro_ under conditions simulating those in the rumen. (e) Do the individual activities, algebraically summed, equal the total activities? This involves the integration of so many factors that its implementation requires computer or similar technology. (f) What factors regulate the ecosystem?

In vitro experiments are indispensable in b, c and d. This paper emphasises _in vitro_ methods for measuring rates of processes in the _in vivo_ rumen ecosystem.

Axenic Cultivation Knowledge of factors concerned in anaerobic isolation of pure cultures has been widely disseminated and needs no further discussion, other than to point out that the axenic animal is a powerful tool that as yet has not been fully exploited. Complete separation of the animal from microbes, with reintroduction of known strains, is of great potential value in ascertaining the exact activities of the microbes in the natural habitat, as well as the reaction to them by the animal.

So far, the investigators using this approach, have not had
available the numbers of axenic animals and key microbial strains
needed to permit a complete analysis. The fact that pure cultures
of rumen microbes grown together form different fermentation
products than when grown apart (1-3) indicates that in vitro
microbial metabolism may differ significantly from that in vivo.
This is particularly true in connection with molecular hydrogen.
Much of the H_2 produced in the rumen is converted to methane,
influencing markedly the formation of other fermentation products.

Pure cultures are indispensable in determining the foods
metabolizable by the microbes and the host but except for extremely
stenotrophic microbes, i.e. microbes using only a few foods, they do
not identify the substrates used in the natural ecosystem. Here,
again, measurements on the total microbiota are essential.

An obvious method for studying the interactions of host and
microbiota is to study their behaviour when separated. This need
not be the separation of each microbe in pure culture, but can be
simply the physical separation of the microbial ecosystem from its
host.

The Zero Time Rate Method Description of the rumen microbial
ecosystem in terms of integrated rates, necessitates measurements of
rates pertinent to the rumen itself. These can be measured in vivo
or, by removal of the ecosystem, they can be measured in vitro.
Removal of the total ecosystem is not usually feasible, and the
investigator must be content with a sample. The objection can be
and is raised that removal of the whole system or of a sample
changes the factors influencing its activity, making in vitro
results of questionable validity. The rationale behind the
development of the zero time rate method accepts the fact that
changes result from changing the environment of a natural ecosystem,
and concentrates on measuring the rate at which the change occurs.

It is not usually feasible to remove the entire gut ecosystem. A sample must be removed from the ecosystem to a physical environment simulating as closely as possible that of the natural ecosystem. It is assumed that drastic changes upon removal cannot occur instantly and that if removal is accomplished without lapse of any time the removed sample will be identical with the natural ecosystem. Such removal is obviously impossible, but if it can be accomplished expeditiously and if there is some assurance that the environment into which it is placed does not differ markedly from the natural one, changes will be gradual rather than cataclysmic.

Evidence of the speed of change can be obtained by measuring the in vitro system at various times after removal of the sample. This allows graphical representation of the parameter studied and estimation from the graph of the rate of change at various times after removal. The slope of the curve at zero time can be estimated graphically by a mirror method (4), and represents the rate of change in both the removed sample and in the ecosystem.

Precautions in Use of the Zero-Time-Rate Method   One of the most fundamental and often overlooked essentials for the success of the method is that the sample must represent, validly not only the liquid, but also the solids fraction of the rument contents. The substrates supporting the fermentation are chiefly those in the undigested fibrous materials. The solids fraction is important also because it harbours about three-fourths of the rumen microbiota. Soluble substrates are quite abundant in many forages but are fermented so rapidly in the rumen that the concentration of soluble unfermented substrates is very small.

Rumen solids are often so abundant that a removed sample has a large surface exposed to the air. This is relatively unimportant insofar as anaerobiosis is concerned, and probably important in other respects, except that the steps usually taken to ensure anaerobiosis can cause a significant drop in temperature. Anaerobiosis is obtained by passing O_2-free gas (CO_2 or CO_2/N_2 in a ratio of 7/3) through the sample container to displace air. The cylinder gases are completely dry, and water evaporates rapidly from the extensive surface area of the sample, causing heat to leave more rapidly than it enters from the water bath. This reduces the initial fermentation rate.

Accumulation of acid and diminution of substrate in the _in vitro_ culture normally slows the rate of fermentation with time, whereas when cooling has occurred the rate increases as the temperature rises. Cooling during oxygen removal can be prevented by passing the cylinder gas through a large-volume evaporator immersed in the water bath and filled with moist cotton or other wettable material to humidify the gas, yet keep it at incubation temperature. In the field, where anaerobic gases may not be available, good results can be obtained by ignoring anaerobiosis, filling the containers quickly, sealing them and immersing in the water bath without any gassing. However, dry ice can often be transported to the field, and used to generate O_2-free CO_2.

Several methods are available to measure changes in rumen parameters during _in vitro_ incubation. The amounts of individual volatile acids or other materials undergoing a change in concentration can be measured by subsampling at various times of incubation. The initial measurement should be made on a subsample taken as soon as possible after removal of the contents from the rumen, because it represents the zero time value. The interval between subsequent measurements depends on the rate of change and the precision of the analysis. The fact that the differences are between rather large values makes accurate analyses essential.

When the individual VFA's are to be measured, the subsamples can be made alkaline enough to stop all microbial growth, and sealed for return to the laboratory for later analysis. Acidified samples usually lose some VFA prior to analysis.

In vitro incubated samples of rumen contents usually show a decline in the rate of production of acetic acid, the most abundant fermentation product, and slower decreases in the rates for propionic and butyric acids. In order to obtain a useful curve at least four points, including the initial analysis, should be obtained. The rate of production of the acids is enough and the analysis sufficiently precise that changes occurring within thirty minutes can be measured reliably. Results obtained with samples incubated longer than that before subsampling are questionable. Not only will the acid production decrease because of the factors previously mentioned, but other processes may increase, e.g. death of some types of microorganisms, growth of others, and microbial decomposition. These processes lead toward further conversion of fermentation acids into carbon dioxide and methane by microorganisms, present in small numbers in the rumen, but multiplying in the incubated sample.

Manometric methods   Manometric methods are useful for measuring the rate of production of the total waste fermentation products, (VFA's), CO_2 and methane. The VFA's react with the bicarbonate to give free CO_2, allowing the total fermentation products to be measured by gas production. This can be accomplished by measuring the increase in gas pressure when the sample is enclosed in a fixed-volume container, or by measurement of the volume of the gas produced at contant pressure (atmospheric). Large (130-ml) round-bottomed flasks can be used in the Warburg-designed instrument for measuring pressure changes, employing mercury in the manometers to accommodate the pressures generated by the large samples needed for reliable representation of the whole rumen. By suitable manipulation (6) it is possible to distinguish the gas pressure due to acid production, to carbon dioxide production and to methane.

Constant pressure measurements are even more easily accomplished than those with constant volume. It is only necessary to transfer the samples as quickly as possible to a water bath, close them with a rubber closure, through which a syringe needle can be inserted to allow escape of gas and leave the container gas at atmospheric pressure. The zero time is then recorded. A syringe, well lubricated (with water or very light oil) is then attached to the needle to collect gases due to fermentation. The amount collected after various time intervals is recorded and plotted to show the rate of production. Frequent measurements can be made, in each instance, reading the gas volume in the vertically held syringe before withdrawing the needle and extruding the gas, prior to taking the next sample. A number of replicates can be measured in this way, and the influence of several factors assessed. It may be helpful to analyze the produced gas for methane, since variables selected for study may modify the relative amounts in which methane is produced.

It is preferable to dilute the sample anaerobically with a balanced salt solution containing 0.5 per-cent sodium bicarbonate at bath temperature in order to allow better mixing. The contents should be mixed before each reading is taken, but continuous shaking is not necessary for equilibration of gas between the gaseous and liquid phases. There seem to be nuclei for gas formation that prevent supersaturation of gas in the liquid.

Examples of in vitro measurements   Measurements of this sort have
been made in order to estimate the rates of production of the
individual VFA's in rumen contents (7,8), to compare the rates of
fermentation in Zebu and European cattle on the same ration (9), to
demonstrate stable foam production in bloating cattle (10), to test
the effect of chlortetracyclines and VFA's added to cattle feed
(11,12), to measure rates of fermentation in the different parts of
the alimentary tract of several wild and domesticated animals (6),
and to estimate the net growth of the rumen population (13).

The net growth rate of the rumen microbiota has been
investigated by an in vitro incubation method according to the
following rationale. It is assumed that the rate of fermentation by
the microbes is directly related to their number and to the
availability of substrate. If excess substrate is provided,
differences in its rate of fermentation can be ascribed to
differences in the number of organisms and, by determining the
change in the rate of fermentation during a short interval of in
vitro incubation, the change in numbers, i.e. the growth rate, can
be estimated. Application of this method to determine microbial
growth rates in a fistulated Jersey heifer fed alfalfa hay (13)
showed a tremendous increase in the rate of fermentation when excess
ground alfalfa plus grain was added to in vitro-incubated samples,
regardless of whether the animal had recently eaten. Substrate was
limiting at all times of the day.

Samples obtained within a few hours after feeding showed
increases in total microbiota activity during an hour of incubation,
whereas at other times a slight decrease was observed. The net
growth rate corresponded fairly well with the values in the
literature for rumen turnover rates, which should equal the
microbial growth rates.

In the experiments studying bloating and non-bloating cattle fed Ladino clover, the initial idea was to detect differences in the rate of the rumen fermentation in the two groups (11). None could be detected, but it was observed that the gas produced by the digesta from animals exhibiting bloat accumulated as foam in the manometric vessel, whereas the gas from the digesta of the non-bloaters did not.

The in vitro experiments with steers fed low levels of chlortetracycline also failed to demonstrate any significant difference between fermentation rates of rumen contents from animals with and without this antibiotic (10). But a change in the antibiotic resistance of the microbiota could be demonstrated by the effect on fermentation rate of the addition of more antibiotic to the fermentation vessels. The controls were inhibited more by added antibiotic than were the rumen samples from the experimental animals receiving the low level of antibiotic; an indication that the composition of the microbiota had changed even though the total fermentation was about the same.

An experiment to test the effect on straw utilization on ration supplementation with valeric and isovaleric acids (12) showed no difference in the fermentation rates of animals with and without the acids, but it was noted that the ration of the supplemented animals was completely consumed soon after administration, whereas that of the controls was barely consumed by the time of the next feeding. These animals were fed a fixed weight of ration. The results on appetite stimulation suggest that ad lib feeding might have shown a favourable effect of the acids on weight gain.

Sampling non-fistulated animals poses problems. In hay or pasture-fed animals it is very difficult to obtain by stomach tube a sample containing a representative proportion of solids. This difficulty was overcome in the study on the relative rates of

fermentation of kikuyu grass by Zebu and European cattle in Kenya
(9). A sample of greater volume than that required for the
fermentation experiments was withdrawn from the animal by stomach
tube, and the solids were collected in coarse gauze. The material
withheld by the cloth was assumed to contain roughly the proportion
of solids characteristic of the whole rumen contents, and was used
as such. Subsequent determinations of dry weights confirmed the
assumption, and there were no significant differences between the
dry weights of the samples from the two cattle species. In each of
six comparisons the Zebu rumen contents exhibited a slightly greater
rate of fermentation than did samples from Bos taurus, the average
difference being about 10 percent, interpreted as indicating a
faster turnover of digesta in the Zebu, correlated with a relatively
smaller rumen.

In some in vitro experiments reliable information on certain
features of the rumen function can be obtained with samples
containing the rumen liquid and its suspended microbes but without
the solids. This is the case when total microbial digestibility of
a feed is determined (5). Omission of rumen solids reduces the
initial dry weight of all samples, and permits use of slightly
larger samples of the feed. The amount of feed added to the vessels
must be sufficiently small to ensure that the fermentation products
do not become inhibitory. Many pure cultures of rumen muralytic
bacteria are inhibited when the concentration of digestible
carbohydrate is greater than 0.15 percent (w/v). These experiments
are of long duration and are most conveniently followed
manometrically.

Rumen liquid, without solids, could also be used in studies of
the affinity (K_s) of rumen methanogenic bacteria for hydrogen
molecular and formate. The effect of various substrate
concentrations on the rate of methanogenesis by a pure culture of
Methanobacterium ruminantium and by rumen liquid was studied, using
a procedure in which the concentration of dissolved H_2 could be
measured (14). The K_s for H_2 was about 10^{-6} M with both the

pure culture and the rumen liquid, whereas the K_s for for formate was greater than 2×10^4 M for the pure culture, but 3×10^5 M for the rumen liquid. This was interpreted as indicating that the methanogen did not use formate in the rumen; instead, it was converted to H_2 and CO_2 by non-methanogenic rumen organisms, and the H_2 then used to reduce CO_2 to methane.

In the above experiments, it was assumed that the variation of the environmental conditions in the experimental vessel from those in the rumen did not affect the fundamental feature of substrate affinities in the bacterial cells. The total rate of the fermentation was not important; rather the relative rates of fermentation with changing substrate concentrations were the critical values.

Advantage of In Vitro Procedures   The acquired instinct of a microbiologist is to isolate pure cultures as the only avenue for obtaining reliable information. But characterization of the rumen microbiota is too time-consuming to be practicable for answering questions about the total population. In many instances the activity of the population as a whole is the factor of concern, and if a clear question is asked, short-term in vitro experiments with the whole ecosystem can be devised to provide answers. An understanding of the several factors concerned in in vitro fermentation may make them more fruitful.

REFERENCES

1. Jayasuriya GCN and Hungate RE. 1959. Lactate conversions in the bovine rumen. Arch. Biochem. Biophys. 82: 274-287.
2. Hungate RE. 1975. The rumen microbial ecosystem. Ann. Rev. Ecology and Systematics 6: 39-64.
3. Moonmaw CR and Hungate RE. 1963. Ethanol conversion in the bovine rumen. J. Bacteriol. 85: 721-722.

150

4. Adams SL and Hungate RE. 1950. Continuous fermentation cycle times: Prediction from growth curve analysis. Indust. Engin. Chem. 42: 1815-1818.

5. Hungate RE. 1966. The Rumen and Its Microbes. New York, Academic Press.

6. Hungate RE, Phillips GD, MacGregor A, Hungate DP and Buechner HK. Microbial fermentation in certain mammals. Science 130: 1192-1194.

7. Carroll EJ and Hungate RE. 1954. The magnitude of the microbial fermentation in the bovine rumen. Appl. Microbiol. 2: 205-214.

8. Hungate RE, Mah RA and Simesen M. 1961. Rates of production of individual volatile fatty acids in the rumen of lactating cows. Appl. Microbiol. 9: 554-561.

9. Hungate RE, Phillips GD, Hungate DP and MacGregor A. 1960. A comparison of the rumen fermentation in European and Zebu cattle. J. Agric. Sci. 54: 196-201.

10. Hungate RE, Fletcher DW, Dougherty RW and Barrentine BF 1955. Microbial activity in the bovine rumen: Its measurement and relation to bloat. Appl. Microbiol. 3: 161-173.

11. Hungate RE, Fletcher DW and Dyer IA. 1955. Effects of chlortetracycline feeding on bovine rumen microorganisms. J. Anim. Sci. 14: 997-1001.

12. Hungate RE and Dyer IA. 1956. Effect of valeric and isovaleric acids on straw utilization by steers. J. Anim. Sci. 15: 485-488.

13. El-Shazly K and Hungate RE. 1965. Fermentation capacity as a measure of net growth of rumen microorganisms. Appl. Microbiol. 13: 62-69.

14. Hungate RE. 1967. Hydrogen as an intermediate in the rumen fermentation. Arch. Mikrobiol. 59: 158-164.

MATHEMATICAL MODELS

P.N. HOBSON

1. INTRODUCTION

In this symposium, a 'model' is a simplified version of some
microbial activity which it is hoped will reproduce a natural
system. This model may be a simplified living system, such as
gnotobiotic lambs where a real animal has a simplified rumen flora
(eg. ref 1) or conversely a tooth in an artificial mouth, with a
natural bacterial flora.

Natural systems are complicated and often sufficiently detailed
analysis, to determine how the system is working, cannot be made;
there are many bacteria, of which the active ones are not known.
There are many uncontrollable external factors which determine
individual changes. The object of the 'living' model is a
simplification of the system to one which can be controlled and
analysed. Variation of parameters then allows reproduction of the
action of a complete natural system.

The natural system may also be described in words and such a
description is a prerequisite for the construction of a living
model. The natural system is, at least initially, not static, but
one which changes with time and may, at death or disintegration,
become static. Verbally one can only describe the progress of this
dynamic system in indefinite terms. If this verbal description can
be translated into mathematical terms, however, then it may be
possible to predict with certainty what the end will be, or the
outcome, should certain controlling parameters or parts of the
system be varied.

Thus, a mathematical model can be predictive, and different parameters can be varied at will to show which are those of greatest importance. Since the model can only work if its terms are correct, it can predict whether sufficiently adequate terms exist to make the system work and indicate what experimental data are lacking in its description. Since natural systems are complicated, however, as with the living model, simplification is necessary otherwise too many unknown terms may exist or the mathematics become too complicated for a solution to be found. It must also be remembered that the mathematical model must be based on experimental fact and biological probability. It is often possible to formulate an equation which will fit a certain set of experimental results. Unless at least some of the constants and variables can be equated with some known biological process and be determined experimentally, the model has no basis in reality and and ceases to be predictive. The system may, therefore, require simplification.

In infection, a situation exists where an initially sterile site becomes infected with a pathogen. Alternatively, an organism may outgrow and become dominant to an existing commensal flora. The bacterium may be a single event contaminant, or it may be a small part of the existing normal flora which, under certain circumstances, attains high numbers.

In order to model the first situation, a knowledge of microbial growth is needed; to model the second, information on how mixed populations maintain steady-state is required.

In a short paper it is impossible to refer to all of the literature or review all aspects of modelling. The work of the author's department is not concerned with infections, as such, but with the functioning of the complex anaerobic bacterial systems of the gut, of the ruminant and of anaerobic digesters. These are dynamic systems which attain a quasi steady-state, mixed population of bacteria, which, while they may be, in some cases using the same substrates, are not directly competing for limiting substrates.

Competition however, and the production of 'antagonistic' substances
may play a part in excluding some organisms from the systems. These
systems may be subject to 'infections' by inoculation from outside,
or by the overgrowth of a bacterium normally present only in
negligible numbers. The second 'infection' results from some change
in, or breakdown of, the controlling factors of the system, and if
the normal system can be modelled, the effects of changes in
controlling factors may also be modelled. In this paper, the
digester and rumen are used to indicate how complex microbial
systems may be modelled in a relatively simple manner and what
information these models may provide. More complex models may then
be constructed by extending the simple model or modifying the
approach.

The digester is a mechanical system in which many of the
parameters influencing microbial growth can be delineated and
controlled, while the rumen is an animal system over which control
is less feasible. Some aspects of earlier mathematical models of
anaerobic digesters and of both mathamatical and gnotobiotic lamb
models of the rumen, were discussed elsewhere (2,3).

Growth and death of bacteria A model of an infection of a sterile
site requires knowledge of bacterial growth. Experiments have shown
that given a sufficient amount of nutrients, bacteria will grow
exponentially in such a way that $N_t = n_o e^{ut}$, where n_o is the
starting number and n_t is the number after time t, and u is a
maximum growth rate. It could then be assumed that infective
bacteria, in a wound, would grow similarly although neither nor u
the exact substrate on which the bacteria are growing is known.
However, if the infective bacterium is known, however, its growth in
a rich broth may be taken as approximating to growth in the wound
and thus a value for u could be determined by experiment.

The model then tells us that at time t after an infection there
will be n_t bacteria in the wound. From this other deductions may
be made e.g. the time taken for the infecting bacterium to produce a
certain amount of toxin. However, this model is too simple and one
obvious fault is that it has no upper limit on n, as time has no
limit. This upper limit may be set by utilisation of substrates in

the wound and so u could be set at a constant rate for a time and then at a declining rate, to zero. Growth of an aerobic bacterium could be limited in rate and extent by access of oxygen. Antibacterial factors in the wound tissue could come into play and result in death of bacteria or their removal from the site. In these situations the system may then be approaching a continuous culture model where bacteria are growing and are washed out of the system.

These effects can be modelled by altering the growth rate of the bacteria. A simple example from our own work, the death and washout of <u>Salmonella anatum</u> in an anaerobic digester (4), although not quite the same situation as been discussed already will illustrate some points. A continuous-flow, stirred-tank digester, by means of a single injection of a large number of salmonellae, simulates a model of a digester, contaminated from faeces of infected pigs, which have then been removed from the herd. The salmonellae do not grow in the mass of digester contents and are actually killed by acids and other factors. This model does not make any direct reference to the digester bacteria: the infection is of a system which produces something toxic to the infecting bacterium.

The digester was running at a retention time of 10 days so, by washout, the numbers in the digester would reduce by the model $n_t = n_o e^{-Dt}$, where $D = 0.1$ d^{-1} (the dilution rate) and t is in days.

The reduction in numbers was greater, however, and could be explained by a death rate j, when $n_t = n_o e^{-(D + j)t}$. thus numbers were reduced from 1.7×10^5 to 0.032×10^5 in 3 days and since D was fixed j was 1.22 d^{-1}. This model, $n_t = n_o e^{-(D + 1.22)t}$, should then be applicable to the digester with salmonella, but operating at different retention times, or to other digesters if the feedstock and temperature were the same as the experimental digester.

Here we have a mechanical system in which all external
parameters can be controlled, so that reasonable values for factors
in the equations may be obtained. In the wound, phagocytosis may be
likened to digester washout, but a value for D would be difficult or
impossible to obtain. The model, moreover, does not describe the
complete course of events after the 'infection'. This model is a
deterministic one indicating that, at all times and in all numbers,
salmonellae washout and die according to the equation. With a large
number of bacteria (1.7×10^5/ml) and with good stirring in the
digester, the bacteria behave as predicted. However, when the
salmonella numbers had dropped to about 10^3/ml (after 3 or 4 days)
their behaviour began to diverge from the model. The numbers of
bacteria found were either greater or fewer than predicted by the
model with small numbers persisting longer (Table 1).

Table 1. Some representative counts showing death and washout of
Salmonella anatum in a pig-waste digester

Time* (days)	Salmonella (per ml)
0	1.67×10^5
3	3.20×10^3
5	1×10^3
7	1.8×10^3
8	12×10^3
9	1.2×10^3
17	3×10^3
24	40
43	30
46	200
53	50
71	10

Death and washout corresponded to the exponential model (see text)
up to 3 or 4 days. On this model all bacteria should have
disappeared by 9 days.

*Days after introduction of Salmonella.

The system had changed from 'determinstic' to 'stochastic' where
the bacteria did not behave as a mass, but as individuals having a
probability of living longer than the mean time, or, possibly,
resisting washing out. The salmonella persisted longer than the
model predicted. A slow growth of some salmonellae was found on the
digester wall, above the liquid level originating from the culture
medium. A search for other factors involved was prompted by the
fact that occasionally some of this dropped off and reinoculated the
liquid.

The simple model for the growth of the wound infection was
deterministic and was predictive of a large inoculum. If the
inoculum contained only a few organisms, there would be a
probability that these would die before they divided, or make only
one or two divisions and then die. Similarly, death or removal of
the bacteria in the wound could follow the same pattern as death of
the salmonellae when low numbers were reached. So the simple model
of the infection must again become more complicated if it is to
describe some infections. It is probable that a wound infection can
be modelled only under particular circumstances.

<u>Mixed bacterial systems</u> The rumen and anaerobic digesters contain
large populations of microorganisms (<u>ca</u>. 10^7 - 10^{10}/ml). The
reactions in a digester treating faecal and other slurries are very
similar to those in the rumen except that there is an added
degradation of long chain fatty acids and conversion of acetic acid
to methane (see, for instance, Hungate, this symposium; refs. 2, 5,
6). The type of digester considered here physicically is similar to
the rumen in that it is a single-stage, stirred tank continuous
culture, with inflow of feedstock and outflow of undegradable feed
residues and bacterial cells.

In the digester the main reactions consist of hydrolysis and
fermentation of fibrous food residues in the faecal feedstock to
acids, hydrogen and carbon dioxide, hydrolysis of lipids and
degradation of long-chain fatty acids to acetic acid. Acetic acid
and hydrogen, plus carbon dioxide are finally converted to methane.
Nitrogenous compounds, principally ammonia, are used in bacterial
cell growth. There are, in addition, other minor metabolic pathways
and interactions. Although the digester, like the rumen, is a

non-sterile system and is open to contamination from the
environment, it can be assumed to have no addition of active
bacteria when it has attained steady-state operation.

Functions of the digester can be modelled in steady-state
operation by considering it as a number independent continuous
cultures, mutually supplying carbonaceous substrate until methane is
formed. The model was first made for a digester treating piggery
waste, and this was well-stirred and fed at five minute intervals.
Since the bacterial population is large, a deterministic model may
be used.

Monod (9) described equations by which the growth of bacteria
could be related to a limiting substrate over a certain range of
concentration. Since then other equations have been suggested as
fitting more exactly the experimental results (10). There are also
Blackman kinetics (11) and a diffusion-enzyme model (12). However,
Monod kinetics seem adequate for most purposes and Herbert, Elsworth
& Telling (13) demonstrated that they could be applied to a pure
culture of bacteria in a continuous-flow culture with a dissolved
substrate. When the system had reached equilibrium at a constant
dilution rate (i.e. 'steady-state'), the residual substrate and
bacterial concentration could be described by differential equations
in which the rates of changes in the system were equated to zero.

The growth of the bacteria is dependent on one limiting
substrate, all others being in excess. At any dilution rate below
that corresponding to a maximum growth rate the concentration of the
residual limiting substrate (s) is $\dfrac{DK_s}{U_m-D}$ where D is dilution rate,
u_m is maximum growth rate of the bacteria on the substrate and
K_s is the substrate concentration which gives half maximum growth
rate. The growth rate up to u_m is dependent on substrate
concentration and is u, where $u = \dfrac{U_mS}{K_s + S} = D.$ The dilution rate
in a stirred-tank culture is flow rate of medium/volume of tank.

The bacteria in an animal-waste digester are limited by an energy source and have excess nitrogen. In the feed to a pig-waste digester, there is non-biodegradable material which passes through the digester unchanged. The first bacterial reaction is hydrolysis and fermentation of the available cellulose and hemicellulose in fibre particles in the feedstock.

Little is known (for example the maximum growth rates and K_s values) about the bacteria concerned in fibre degradation in digesters, except that there are many species (14, 15). However, because the digester is in a steady-state, the population can be assumed to behave as a pure culture. Computer prediction then indicates that the residual solids (and so the solids degraded) in a digester in a steady-state at different dilution rates, can be described by the Monod-Herbert model with reasonable values of u_m and K_s. K_s is a weight related to surface area of the fibres available for bacterial colonisation and not a concentration of substrate in solution.

However, it was shown experimentally that what should have been a smooth curve of solids degraded against D had a kink in it. This was modelled by assuming two solid substrates, of different particle size but not chemical composition, with different values for u_m and K_s. The more resistant particles cease to be degraded at about 7 or 8 days retention time (1/D) and the more easily degradable particles at about 3 or 4 days. Although this separation into two particle sizes is a simplification (as there is a range of particle sizes in the waste) it has some experimental basis (8).

Thus the solids degradation in a pig-waste digester can be modelled by assuming that a very complex system behaves in mass as a simple one. One property of a model is that it should be tested under conditions different from those used to establish it. Applying to the u_m values an equation for change in u_m with temperature developed from observations on bacteria in other systems (16) the model was used to predict the gas observations of the behaviour of the digester at different temperatures and explained an anomaly in experimental gas productions. The model also fits cattle-waste digestions, although here the values of u_m and K_s and the proportions of the two solids fractions have to be changed. This is reasonable, because although the chemical composition is similar, the particle sizes in pig and cattle faeces differ.

The further stages of the digestion, conversion of acids and hydrogen to methane is somewhat simpler. Although numbers of species of bacteria are concerned in each reaction, there is only one, dissolved, substrate for each. Values for u_m and K_s can be obtained from laboratory cultures and these values describe quite well the residual acetic acid and hydrogen in cattle- and pig-waste digesters. The same values for constants are used for each system since the dissolved substrates are of the same composition in each and, so far as is known, the bacteria are the same.

Ammonia can inhibit digestion and from experimental work an equation involving ammonia concentration and u_m can be obtained and applied to u_m in the equations for acid and hydrogen utilization in the digesters. This reproduces the behaviour of pig-waste digesters with high feedstock ammonia concentrations and shows how methane production is inhibited and hydrogen and acetate builds up. Other inhibitions can be similarly modelled.

The model assumes a constant, optimum, pH for the digester. Changes in pH can affect growth rates, and may reverse relative growth rates so that a 'foreign' bacterium becomes dominant, as in rumen lactic acidosis (17).

It will have been noted that while the model describes the results of bacterial growth, in substrates metabolised and products formed, it does not make any reference to bacterial cell production during the digestion process. In theory this is easy to calculate since it involves only a knowledge of substrates used (which is defined in the model) and a yield factor (Y) of grams of cells produced per unit weight of substrate utilized. However, experiments have shown that Y is not a constant, particularly with these anaerobic bacteria, but is proportional to growth rate over a certain range. At the very low growth rates which, overall, must apertain in anaerobic digesters, the dependence of Y on u (or D) becomes uncertain (e.g. 18, 19). The death rate of bacteria becomes much higher than at rates nearer maximum (20). There is little or no experimental data on values for Y in anaerobes, hence estimates of Y would have little factual basis. Further, the complexity of the digester flora, as a whole, is so great that there is no way of validating the model on present experimental evidence.

The model assumes that inflow of feed is completely continuous and it can reproduce the working of a digester system because although the digester is fed at discreet intervals, often of some hours, these are short compared with the retention times of the microbes and feed, and with the overall doubling times of the bacteria. For experimental reasons the determined steady-state concentration of substrates are averages of many measurements over weeks or months, and these agree with the model. The steady-state model could also reproduce the average feed conversions in an animal system such as the rumen, if the animal were fed at a few minute intervals with a few grams of feed. This gives time factors analagous to the digester system but 'compressed' into hours and minutes rather than days, and can be experimentally obtained with animals trained to eat continuously from feed presented in small amounts by a conveyor system. The model cannot reproduce relatively short-term variations in microbial activity and the average values for substrates remaining, etc., have greater deviations from actual values at any particular time as intervals between feeds and amounts fed become greater in relation to system turnover time. The steady-state system also has to attain this condition from some other steady-state, or from an initially sterile state, and the model cannot simulate this.

For 'quasi' steady-state systems or ones approaching steady-state, a dynamic model is needed. The model may, in the first instance, like the steady-state model, consider only substrate metabolism without production of bacteria. An input of substrate and its degradation and washout, can be considered as occurring exponentially over a period before the next addition of substrate. Residual substrate from the first addition, is added to the second addition and both are degraded and washed out, and so on. In effect this becomes a series of batch microbial cultures superimposed on a continuous-flow system.

When a degradation rate of substrate rather than a growth rate of bacteria is considered as a first approximation the two can be considered as related. The degradation rate may be a constant. For example when substrate inputs are high, the substrate concentration will maintain the bacteria at near maximum growth rate; in contrast with low substrate inputs, degradation rate can be made to vary with the substrate concentration, in the same way as does the growth rate previously discussed.

In this type of model, with a number of repeated feedings from starting the digester, changing animal diet, or introducing to the anaerobic digester feed, at start-time intervals will produce a system approaching, at infinite time, steady-state values of residual substrate with substrate degradation and wash-out between each feed.

The steady state of the first model represents a state where, as substrate enters the culture, it is metabolised and the growth rate of the bacteria increases for a time. Then, if the substrate concentration drops below steady-state level the growth rate decreases and substrate builds up. So the culture is actually oscillating, but in the model oscillations are infinitely small. The dynamic model for substrate degradation can be made to come to the steady-state model residual substrate concentration at a particular dilution rate and oscillate about this concentration by making a sudden increase in substrate concentration 'trigger-off' a high degradation rate. Below some substrate level, near the steady-state concentration, the rate depends on the concentration in the same way as growth rate. The high rate of degradation is uncoupled from bacterial growth and while the build up of the bacterial population must follow the substrate degradation, the 'uncoupling' presents another difficulty in modelling the yield of bacteria. This model is still being investigated, but it seems to represent a phenomenon similar to that observed in a continuous

culture of _Aerobacter aerogenes_ by Neijssel & Tempest (21) and
called by them 'energy-spill' metabolism. Walker & Nader (22) also
found that in the period after consumption of a feed fermentation in
the rumen was not coupled to microbial cell synthesis, but ATP
energy was either 'wasted' or used in synthesis of storage
polysaccharide. The model has been tested for solids degradation in
the anaerobic digester with some different dilution rates and
intervals between feeds. At the limit, when feed additions are
infinitesimally small and at infinitesimal time intervals, it
becomes the steady-state model.

What has been attempted in this section of a short paper is to
show that complex microbial systems may be modelled in relatively
simple and yet biologically probable ways and that these models can
not only describe the systems but also show how the normal systems
may react to changes in feed and environment. Thus it may be
possible to predict under what conditions the system will be liable
to takeover by an infective bacterium.

While these models have described the results of bacterial
metabolism, they have said, for the reasons given, little or nothing
about the growth of the bacterial cells. Assigning values to
factors is a major problem in modelling complex microbial systems
such as the intestinal tract. Computer iteration may define a
value. In the case of the 'overspill metabolism' model above, only
certain rates of uncoupled substrate degradation will bring the
starting up digester to the required steady states. However,
equating these with experimental results is, as in other cases,
difficult or impossible. The active bacteria in the natural mixture
may not have been isolated, or the relative importance of isolates
in the natural population may be unknown. Even if the active
bacteria are known, metabolic rates in the natural, mixed culture
may differ from those determined in pure cultures on substrates that
are probably modified natural products. One way of testing the
basic principles of, for instance, a simple model rumen is that used
by the author in some unpublished work. The model was compared to
data on rumen function in a sheep fed automatically at fixed
intervals on completely 'synthetic' feeds (prepared cellulose,

starch, etc.) (23). The analysis of the feed degradation and microbial production was thus more precise than in a normally-fed animal, and data from cultures of representative cellulolytic, amylolytic, etc., rumen bacteria could be used in the model, or used to compare with values required to make the model reproduce the rumen function.

More complex models of natural systems have been proposed, for instance for the rumen by Baldwin and co-workers who have attempted to make the microbial system less of a 'black box', by putting in equations for production of individual volatile fatty acids, and for other metabolic pathways. They have used a mixture of data from pure cultures and average data from many feeding experiments with animals to obtain values for terms, but lack of suitable data is, again, a major problem and, overall, the models have produced only relatively simple results. This has all been discussed in more detail elsewhere (3).

CONCLUSION

Modelling of natural microbial communities is difficult even when the environment of the community can be defined in an apparatus in vitro. In vivo, the ill-defined environment can present further problems. Nevertheless, mathematical modelling can help in explaining the behaviour of microbial systems and in suggesting where further experimental work is needed.

REFERENCES

1. Hobson PN, Mann SO and Steward CS. 1981. Growth and rumen function in gnotobiotic lambs fed on starch diets. J. gen. Microbiol. 126, 219-230.
2. Hobson PN, Bousfield S and Summers R. 1974. The anaerobic digestion of organic matter. Crit. Rev. Environ. Control 4, 131-191.
3. Hobson PN and Wallace RJ. 1982. Microbial ecology and activities in the rumen, parts 1 and 2. Crit. Rev. Microbiol. 9, 165-225, 253-320.
4. Summers R, Bousfield S and Hobson PN. 1980. In Anaerobic Digestion, ed. D.A. Stafford et al., London, Applied Science Publishers, pp. 409-414.
5. Hobson PN, Bousfield S and Summers R. 1981. Methane Production from Agricultural and Domestic Wastes. London, Applied Science Publishers.

164

6. Hobson PN. 1981. Microbial pathways and interactions in the anaerobic treatment process. In Mixed Culture Fermentations, ed. M.E. Bushell and J.H. Slater. London, Academic Press, pp. 53-79.
7. Hobson PN and McDonald I. 1980. Methane production from acids in piggery waste digesters. J. Chem. Tech. Biotech. 30. 405-408.
8. Hobson PN. 1983. The kinetics of anaerobic digestion of farm wastes. J. Chem. Tech. Biotech. 33B, 1-20.
9. Monod J. 1942. Richerches sur la Croissance des Cultures Bacteriennes. Paris, Hermann et Cie.
10. Powell EO. 1967. The growth rate of microorganisms as a function of substrate concentration. In, Microbial Physiology and Continuous Culture. Ed. E.O. Powell, et al. London, H.M.S.O. pp. 34-55.
11. Condrey RE. 1982. The chemostat and Blackman Kinetics. Biotech. Bioeng. 24, 1705-1709.
12. Koch AL. 1982. Multistep kinetics: choice of models for the growth of bacteria. J. theor. Biol. 98, 401-417.
13. Herbert D, Elsworth R and Telling RC. 1956. The continuous culture of bacteria; a theoretical and experimental study. J. gen. Microbiol. 14, 601-622.
14. Hobson PN and Shaw BG. 1974. The bacterial population of piggery waste anaerobic digesters. Water Res. 8, 507-516.
15. Sharma VK. 1983. The isolation and characterisation of cellulolytic bacteria from a cattle waste anaerobic digester. Ph.D. thesis, Aberdeen.
16. Ratkowsky DA, Olley J, McMechin TA and Ball A. 1982. Relationship between temperature and growth rate of bacterial cultures. J. Bacteriol. 149, 1-5.
17. Hobson PN and Steward CS. 1970. Growth of two rumen bacteria in mixed culture. J. gen. Microbiol. 63, XI.
18. Hobson PN. 1965. Continuous culture of some anaerobic and facultative rumen bacteria. J. gen. Microbiol. 38, 167-180.
19. Hobson PN and Summers R. 1967. The continuous culture of anaerobic bacteria. J. gen. Microbiol. 47, 53-65.
20. Tempest DW, Herbert D and Phipps PJ. 1967. Studies on the growth of Aerobacter aerogenes at low dilution rate in a chemostat. In, Microbial Physiology and Continuous Culture, Ed. E.O. Powell London, H.M.S.O.
21. Neijssel OM and Tempest DW. 1976. The role of energy-spilling reactions in the growth of Klebsiella aerogenes NCTC418 in aerobic chemostat culture. Arch. Microbiol. 110, 305-311.
22. Walker DJ and Nader CJ. 1970. Rumen microbial protein synthesis in relation to energy supply: diurnal variation with once-daily feeding. Aust. J. Agric. Res. 21, 747-754.
23. Hume ID, Moir RJ and Somers M. 1970. Synthesis of microbial protein in the rumen. 1. Influence of the level of nitrogen intake. Aust. J. Agric. Res. 21, 283-296.

THE APPLICATION OF CONTINUOUS CULTURE TECHNIQUES TO THE STUDY OF
ORAL ANAEROBES

ALISA S. MCKEE, ANN S. McDERMID, P.D. MARSH AND D.C. ELLWOOD

The oral cavity supports a great diversity of micro-organisms,
ranging from aerobes to strict anaerobes. The tooth surface, saliva
and soft tissues each contain their own commensal flora. Dental
plaque, the microbial community on the tooth surface, has been the
subject of much investigation because of its role in the aetiology
of both dental caries and periodontal disease. Two different
approaches have been used to simulate the oral environment in an
attempt to understand microbial behaviour in the mouth: one of
these is the artificial mouth, the other is the chemostat.

THE ARTIFICIAL MOUTH

The artificial mouth comprises a tooth with pH and
reduction-oxidation (red-ox) electrodes attached to the tooth
surface, by drilling holes through the longitudinal axis of the
tooth (1). This model system can then be enclosed and sterilised.
An opening above the tooth permits media, bacterial culture, saliva,
etc. to be dropped aseptically over the tooth surface; waste liquid
is then collected in an effluent reservoir below. Once artificial
plaque has developed, carbohydrates or inhibitors such as fluoride
can then be applied to the tooth surface and the effect on the pH
and red-ox potential of the plaque observed. Sampling the flora
can be done by removing plaque from the tooth surface, or by
withdrawing a tooth segment from a specially designed multiple tooth
unit (2). Others (3) samples the effluent as they found this
reflected gross changes in the plaque flora, but its composition was
not identical to that found at the tooth surface. Mixed cultures,
as well as monocultures, have been investigated and the persistence
of anaerobic bacteria recorded, indicating bacterial interaction, in

which the red-ox potential was lowered sufficiently by microaeorophilic species to enable strict anaerobes to grow in a similar manner to that found in the mouth (3). The addition of sucrose to this community caused the pH to fall, the red-ox to rise, the anaerobes to disappear and the streptococci to predominate. Using this model system, it has been possible to imitate some of the in vivo plaque studies. Inhibitors such as fluoride and chlorhexidine reduced the acid production by plaque bacteria. In this way the effects of dietary carbohydrates or sugar substitutes on the production of plaque acids can be studied. The artificial mouth as a model of the tooth in the oral cavity is successful in its ability to monitor the changes in pH and red-ox potential of plaque at the tooth surface in response to different stimuli. Where the artificial mouth falls short is that it is unable to control the bacterial growth. This is one of the main attributes of the second method of studying the oral community, the use of continuous culture.

THE CHEMOSTAT

The chemostat provides a unique way of studying phenotypic change in a controlled environment, in response to various stimuli. It is a vessel containing a continuously stirred culture in which a series of controls maintain constant pH, temperature, and other chosen environmental factors. Fresh media is pumped into this vessel at a constant flow rate (f). A weir in the pot maintains a constant culture volume (v) and enables continuous effluent collection into a receiver. The medium contains an excess of all essential nutrients except one, which is then growth limiting. Any essential nutrient can be chosen to limit growth, but most studies cited here use glucose to limit the carbon source, while glucose-excess conditions are a device used to limit some nitrogenous material, often cysteine or arginine. By altering the flow rate (f) of the fresh media entering the culture vessel, one can determine the rate of bacterial growth. Dilution rate (D) is the volume of media entering the chemostat per hour (h) per volume (v) of the culture in the vessel.

D = f/v where f = flow of media in millilitres (ml) per hour.

v = volume of the chemostat culture in ml.

The mean generation time (MGT) of an organism growing in continuous culture is calculated by the equation

$$MGT = \ln_2 D^{-1} \quad (\ln_2 = 0.693)$$

Dilution rates of $0.05h^{-1}$ and $0.5h^{-1}$ are, therefore, equivalent to MGT of 14h and 1.4h respectively.

The progression from the simple chemostat to gradient systems and multistage systems in which a series of chemostats are linked together were discussed both theoretically and practically by Herbert (4). The effect of bidirectional flow of different solutes on the physiology of the cells has been studies by Cooper & Copeland (5) and Lovitt and Wimpenny (6). For a recent general review of continuous culture studies see Calcott (7). Veilleux & Rowland (8) used a 2-stage chemostat system to model the rat intestine. Some of the effluent from the first chemostat was pumped into a second vessel which was growing under different conditions. In this way a different population was selected and maintained.

One of the main attributes of continuous culture is that the cells constitute a homogenous liquid culture. This controlled homogeneity is rarely found in natural ecosystems where the presence of many different surfaces must affect the development of the community. Replaceable surfaces were incorporated into a chemostat in order to study the bacterial communities of river and estuarine samples (9,10). Significantly the bacterial community found on these surfaces was different from those in the liquid culture.

ORAL CHEMOSTAT STUDIES

In the oral field most of the continuous culture studies have been conducted using monocultures to study the physiology of the organisms cultured under different growth conditions. Justification of the use of the chemostat in this way is provided by comparison of the fermentation products of oral streptococci found in vitro with those detected in dental plaque before and after meals in vivo. Batch culture studies suggested that oral streptococci were homofermentative with respect to lactic acid. However, chemostat studies have shown that when S. mutans and S. sanguis are grown glucose-limited or at slow growth rates, the conversion of glucose to lactic acid is low. The predominant products of metabolism are formic acid, acetic acid and ethanol, homolactic acid fermentation being seen only under glucose-excess conditions or under glucose-limitation at fast dilution rates (11,12,13). Similarly, a glucose-limited chemostat intermittently pulsed with glucose to simulate in vivo conditions, accumulated lactic acid only after each carbohydrate pulse (14). The acids present in plaque show similar variation, little lactic acid was found from overnight starved plaque of monkeys (15), rats (16) and of man (17), whereas lactic acid is the predominant acid in human dental plaque following the ingestion of dietary carbohydrates (17,18,19). This implies that the regulatory mechanisms imposed on the cells in the chemostat are similar to those operating in dental plaque.

Changes in concentrations of glucose, amino acids and in the pH of the growth medium have been used to study the induction of enzymes and sugar transport systems as well as the changing pattern of fermentation products together with the sensitivity to inhibitors used in preventative dentistry such as fluoride (20-22).

ANAEROBIC MONOCULTURE

B. gingivalis (strain W50) has been grown anaerobically in continuous culture in our laboratory. This organism was chosen for further study because of its known pathogenic potential in periodontal disease (23) and because a considerable amount is already known about its chemical composition (24). In addition van Steenberger (25) using a pathogenicity test in mice showed that only B. gingivalis strains produced an invasive spreading inflammatory response which led to mouse death. All the other black pigmenting Bacteroides strains such as ss melaninogenicus, ss intermedium, and B. asaccharolyticus (the gut strains) produced a more localised response around the injection site. Our preliminary results using chemostat-grown cells indicate the importance of haemin as an essential growth factor.

1. Cells grown in BM + haemin (5 ug/ml) + vitamin K$_1$ (1 ug/ml)
    were pathogenic in mice (26).

2. Cells grown in BM + haemin (vitamin K$_1$ absent) were still
    pathogenic.

3. Cells grown in BM + haemin (0.5 µg/ml) had reduced pathogenicity.

4. Cells grown in BM without haemin (with or without vitamin K$_1$)
    were unable to grow and were washed out of the chemostat.

The animal model for virulence testing enables the state of the
chemostat cells grown under different growth conditions to be
correlated not only with loss or gain of structures such as capsules
(27), change in chemical composition, or extracellular product, but
also with their pathogenic potential.

BINARY CULTURE

Although most oral bacteria produce acid from carbohydrate,
Veillonella sp does not, although it can metabolise lactate to
propionic and acetic acids. In a mixed continuous culture with
Veillonella and Streptococcus mutans, Mikx and van der Hoeven (13)
were able to demonstrate that secondary feeding was taking place,
the glucose in the medium being fermented by S. mutans to lactic
acid which was then being converted to propionic and acetic acids by
the Veillonella. Fewer carious lesions were observed in rats
infected with either S. mutans or S. sanguis and Veillonella, than
in animals infected with either Streptococcus alone. By converting
lactic acid to weaker acids Veillonella species are believed to
reduce the caries-potential of the oral populations. This
relationship was originally considered to be of benefit only to the
lactate consumer, but recent studies have shown that lactate efflux
from the bacterial cell is an energy-generating process (28,29).
The maintenance of a favourable gradient for lactate production by
the presence of bacteria utilising this lactate could benefit both
the consuming and producing organisms (30,31).

PLAQUE MIXED CULTURE

In a plaque study (32) the influence of growth rate and nutrient limitation on the microbial composition of dental plaque was examined. Freshly collected plaque was homogenised and inoculated simultaneously into a glucose-limited and glucose-excess chemostat, with the following results:

1. Many different organisms were able to grow together at dilution rates ranging from 0.05 to 0.6.

2. Some organisms including L. casei and S. mitior were isolated from every sample, while other species, such as B. melaninogenicus and Fusobacterium nucleatum, were only present in the glucose-limited chemostat.

3. A higher percentage of extracellular polysaccharide (EPS) producers were isolated from the glucose-excess chemostat throughout the range of dilution rates. Under glucose-limited conditions only $D = 0.6 \text{ h}^{-1}$ contained an appreciable number of EPS-producing streptococci.

4. The glucose-limited chemostat always contained a more diverse community and gave higher cell yields than the glucose-excess chemostat. Lower terminal pH values were always obtained from washed glucose-excess cells after a pulse of a carbohydrate. This is in contrast to monocultures where the glucose-limited cells always gave the lower terminal pH value.

5. Wall growth, examined at the end of the run, was, in general, less complex than its respective liquid culture. Streptococci, though not EPS producers, were the predominant organisms recovered from the glucose-limited walls, whereas lactobacilli predominated on the glucose-excess walls.

The chemostat community was never identical to the original inoculum. Its metabolic activity however was similar to natural plaque in that lactic acid was the major end product of carbohydrate metabolism under glucose-excess conditions, in contrast to the mixture of acids found under glucose-limited conditions. In vivo studies examining starved overnight plaque fluid (glucose-limiting) and plaque fluid after the ingestion of dietary carbohydrate (glucose-excess) showed similar patterns of acids (17,18).

DEFINED MIXED CULTURE

In an attempt to simplify and, therefore, understand some of the interactions taking place in the oral community a similar mixed culture study was performed using 9 defined oral organisms. The strains used were A. viscosus WUV627; S. mutans (Streptomycin resistant and EPS+) ATCC2-27351; S. sanguis (EPS+) NCTC 7865; S. mitior (EPS-) 7864; L. casei AC413; B. melaninogenicus ss intermedium T588; F. nucleatum NCTC 10953; V. alkalescens ATCC 17745; and a Neisseria species A1078/79. All strains were grown in batch culture, the broths mixed together and a glucose-limited and glucose-excess chemostat inoculated. The chemostats were then adjusted to give a media flow rate corresponding to D = 0.05 h^{-1}, and at pH 7.0. The gas phase used was 5% carbon dioxide in nitrogen, the temperature 37°C and the culture volume 600 ml. In order to assist the more slowly growing strains to establish, 2 further similar inoculations were made on days 4 and 9. Daily viable counts were performed for the first 15 days, after which cell counts were performed 2 to 3 times a week (for 2 weeks from the glucose-excess chemostat and for 6 weeks from the glucose-limited chemostat).

Figure 1 is a simplified graph of the viable counts from the two chemostats during the initial 14 day period.

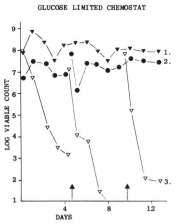
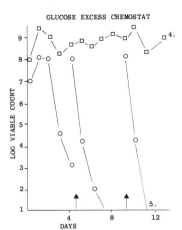

GLUCOSE LIMITED CHEMOSTAT   GLUCOSE EXCESS CHEMOSTAT

1. V. ALKALESCENS, S. MITIOR, L. CASEI
2. F. NUCLEATUM AND B. MELANINOGENICUS
3. NEISSERIA SP.

4. V. ALKALESCENS AND L. CASEI
5. B. MELANINOGENICUS
↑ REINOCULATION

There was a considerable difference in the response from the same inoculum when grown under different conditions. The glucose limited chemostat demonstrated that reinoculation permitted Neisseria, fig. 1 graph 3, which seemed to be lost, to reappear and be maintained at a low level throughout. All species inoculated grew under glucose-limitation, whereas S. mutans, Neisseria and B. melaninogenicus were eliminated from the glucose-excess chemostat. The species which constituted the highest proportion of the viable counts, initially, (figure 1, graphs 1 and 4) retained their dominance throughout. All other species present constituted less than 1% of their respective total counts under "steady state" conditions (Table 1, D).

As a film of growth had developed on the walls of both chemostats during the run, samples from 3 different zones were examined: (A) was above the liquid, (B) was below and (C) was at the liquid-gas interphase (Table 1).

TABLE 1.   MICROBIAL COMPOSITION OF WALL GROWTH

BACTERIAL SPECIES	PERCENTAGE OF TOTAL VIABLE COUNT							
	GLUCOSE LIMITED CHEMOSTAT				GLUCOSE EXCESS CHEMOSTAT			
	A	B	C	D	A	B	C	D
L.CASEI	14	65	5	18	97	24	40	37
S.SANGUIS	0.6	2	17	0.5	0.5	+	0.5	0.3
S.MUTANS	ND	ND	ND	+	ND	ND	ND	ND
S.MITIOR	II	8	23	32	ND	ND	ND	0.6
V.ALKALESCENS	32	9	6	40	3	76	60	61
NEISSERIA SP.	28	1	17	+	ND	ND	ND	ND
B.MELANINOGENICUS	10	11	0.9	5	ND	ND	ND	ND
F.NUCLEATUM	1	4	26	4	ND	+	+	0.3
A.VISCOSUS	3	ND	6	0.6	+	+	0.2	0.4

A is WALL GROWTH REMOVED FROM AREA 1 INCH ABOVE LIQUID SURFACE
B is "   "   "   "   " 1 INCH BELOW   "   "
C is "   "   "   " INTERPHASE OF LIQUID AND GAS
D is from LIQUID CULTURE (FOR COMPARISON)
+ REPRESENTS < 0.1 %
ND is NOT DETECTED

The glucose-excess chemostat B and C zones gave similar results to the liquid culture D, except for the absence of S. mitior. L. casei constituted a very high proportion of the viable count above the liquid where pH control would be minimal, but other species were still present in low numbers. Each zone from the glucose limited walls grew all strains except S. mutans. The interphase zone C showed unusually high viable counts of F. nucleatum, S. sanguis and Neisseria. In contrast to the glucose-excess chemostat, the glucose-limited wall growth zone A, above the liquid, grew all species (Except S. mutans). This suggests that, in the absence of glucose and, therefore acid, the community is able to tolerate, if not use, the metabolic products of one another. A much more diverse number of species is thus retained compared with that established under glucose-excess conditions where acid (predominately lactic acid) could lower the pH to below pH 5.0.

Thus these 2 fermenters, seeded with identical inocula, produced quite different stable populations. The glucose-limited conditions sustained a more varied flora than that found under conditions of glucose-excess. Wall growth though uncontrolled, provided a hard surface for attachment, thus adding another dimension to chemostat growth. Like its liquid culture, the glucose-limited wall growth as found in its corresponding liquid culture, was able to maintain a greater species diversity than that exhibited under glucose-excess conditions.

The chemostat has shown how changes in the environment can bring about phenotypic change which may alter the physiology of the cells. There is still much work to be done in the field of oral microbiology with both single and mixed cultures. Modifications in design, such as the incorporation of removable surfaces in the chemostat, would increase the scope of the modelling, and also extend the possibility of imitating the behaviour of the natural environment.

1. Russell C, Coulter WA. 1975. Continuous monitoring of pH and Eh in bacterial plaque grown in an artificial mouth. Appl. Microbiol. 29, 141-144.
2. Dibden et al. 1976. An apparatus for the continuous culture of micro-organisms on solid surfaces with special reference to dental plaque. J. Appl. Bacteriol. 40, 261-268.

174

3. Coulter WA and Russell C. 1976. pH and Eh in single and mixed culture bacterial plaque in an artificial mouth. J. Appl. Bacteriol. 40, 73-87.

4. Herbert D. 1964. Multistage continuous culture in continuous culture of microorganisms. Proc. 2nd Symp. Prague. Ed. I Malek, K Beran and J Hospodka. Prague, Publishing House Czechoslovak Academy of Science, 1964, 23.

5. Cooper DG and Copeland BJ. 1973. Responses of a continuous series of estuarine microecosystems to point-source input variations Ecol. monogr. 43, 213-236.

6. Lovitt RW and Wimpenny JWT. 1981. The gravostat: a bidirectional compound chemostat and its application in microbiological research. J. Gen. Microbiol. 127, 261-268.

7. Calcott PH. 1981. Continuous cultures of cells. Vol 1. Ed. PH Calcott. CRC Press Inc.

8. Vailleux BG and Rowland I. 1981. Simulation of the Rat Intestinal Ecosystem using a two-stage continuous culture system. J. Gen. Microbiol. 123, 103-115.

9. Brown CM et al 1977. Growth of bacteria at surfaces: influence of nutrient limitation. FEMS Microbiol. Lett. 1, 163-166.

10. Wardell JN, et al. 1980. A continuous culture study of the attachment of bacteria to surfaces. In microbial Adhesion to Surfaces, pp 221-230. Ed. RCW Berkeley et al. Chichester, Ellis Horwood.

11. Ellwood DC, et al. 1974. Growth of Streptococcus mutans in a chemostat. Arch. Oral Biol. 19, 659-665.

12. Carlsson J and Griffith CJ. 1974. Fermentation products and bacterial yields in glucose-limited and nitrogen-limited cultures of streptococci. Arch. Oral Biol. 19, 1105-1109.

13. Mikx FHM and van der Hoeven 1975. Symbiosis of Streptococcus mutans and Veillonella alkalescens in mixed continuous culture. Arch. Oral Biol. 20, 407-410.

14. Cooney CL. et al. 1976. Growth of Enterobacter aerogenes in a chemostat with double nutrient limitations. Appl. Environ. Microbiol. 31, 91-98.

15. Cole MF, et al. 1978. The effect of pyridoxine, phytate and invert sugar on production of plaque acids in situ in the monkey (M. fascicularis). Caries Res. 12, 190-201.

16. Van der Hoeven et al. 1978. Symbiotic relationship of Veillonella alkalescens and Streptococcus mutans in dental plaque in gnotobiotic rats. Caries Res. 12, 142-147.

17. Geddes D.A.M. 1975. Acids produced by human dental plaque metabolism in situ. Caries Res. 9, 98-109.

18. Geddes DAM. 1972. The production of L(+) and L(-) lactic acid and volatile acids by human dental plaque and the effect of plaque buffering and acidic strength of pH. Arch. Oral Biol. 17, 537-545.

19. Gilmour MN, et al. 1976. The C_1-C_4 monocarboxylic and lactic acids in dental plaques before and after exposure to sucrose in vivo. In Microbial Aspects of Dental Caries 1, pp 539-556 . Ed. HM Stiles, WJ Loesche and TC O'Brien. Washington DC, Information Retrieval.

20. Ellwood DC and Hunter JR. 1976. The mouth as a chemostat. In Continuous Culture 6. Applications and New Fields, Ed. ACR Dean, DC Ellwood, GC Evans and J Melling. Chichester, Ellis Horwood.

21. Ellwood DC et al. 1979. Effect of growth rate and glucose concentration on the activity of the phosphoenolpyruvate phosphotransferase system in Streptococcus mutans grown in continuous culture. Infect. Immun. 23, 224-231.
22. Hamilton I and Ellwood DC. 1978. Effects of fluoride on carbohydrate metabolism by washed cells of Streptococcus mutans grown in various pH values in a chemostat. Infect. Immun. 19, 434-442.
23. Slots J. 1979. Subgingival microflora and periodontal disease. J. Clin. Periodontol. 6, 351-382.
24. Shah HN and Collins MD. 1980. Fatty acid and isoprenoid quinone composition in the classification of Bacteroides melaninogenicus and related taxa. J. Appl. Bacteriol. 48, 75-87.
25. Van Steenberger TJM. et al. 1982. Virulence of black pigmented Bacteroides. Strains from periodontal pockets and other sites in experimentally induced skin lesions in mice. J. Periodontol Res. 17, 41-49.
26. Shah HN. et al. 1976. Comparison of the biochemical properties of Bacteroides melaninogenicus from human dental plaque and other sites. J. Appl. Bacteriol. 41, 473-492.
27. Handley PS and Tipler L.S. 1983. In press.
28. Michels PAM, et al. 1979. Generation of an electrochemical proton gradient in bacteria by the excretion of metabolic end-products. FEMS Microbiol. Lett. 5, 357-364.
29. Otto R, et al. 1980. Generation of an electrochemical proton gradient in Streptococcus cremoris by lactate efflux. Proc. Nat. Acad. Sci. USA, 77, 5502-5505.
30. Konigs WN and Veldkamp H. 1980. Phenotypic responses to environmental change. In Contemporary Microbial Ecology, 161-191. Ed. DC Ellwood, JN Hedger, MJ Latham, JM Lynch and JH Slater. London, Academic Press.
31. Ellwood DC. et al. 1982. Surface associated growth. New dimensions in Microbiology. Mixed substrate, mixed cultures and microbial communities pp 71-86. Ed. JP Quayle and AT Bull. London, The Royal Society.
32. Marsh PD, et al. 1983. The influence of growth rate and nutrient limitation on the microbial composition and biochemical properties of a mixed culture of oral bacteria grown in a chemostat. J. Gen Microbiol. 129, 755-770.

IN VITRO MODELS OF THE MAMMALIAN CAECUM AND COLON

I.R. ROWLAND

1. INTRODUCTION

The indigenous microflora of the mammalian gastrointestinal tract influences significantly the anatomical, physiological and immunological characteristics of its host (1,2). It is important therefore to understand the ecological mechanisms governing interactions between the bacteria and host and amongst the bacteria themselves and also to study the contribution of the gut flora to the metabolism of ingested compounds and host secretions. The relationships between a few gut organisms has been studied in vitro (3) and by specifically colonizing germ-free rodents (4), but the interspecific mechanisms observed in such simple systems may not be relevant to the more complex environment of the gut. The study of the ecology of the microflora and its metabolic activity in vitro is complicated by the difficulties of cultivating the flora as a complex mixed culture. The conventional cultural techniques, which employ batch or 'closed' cultures, remove most of the biotic and abiotic constraints in the in-vivo ecosystem. This can result in a distortion of the proportions of the components of the flora, so that metabolism and ecological interactions in such cultures may not be representative of those found in the gut.

A potentially more useful and effective method of culturing and modelling the gut microflora is continuous culture, which has been used successfully to model the rumen ecosystem (5,6). In a continuous culture system, the bacteria are suspended in a medium at a constant volume and at or near to a steady state of growth which is established by continuous addition of fresh growth medium and continuous removal of an equal volume of the culture. This system may be considered roughly analogous to the gut ecosystem. Nutrients, in the form of ingested food components and host secretions, are supplied to a population of microorganisms in an approximately steady state of growth, since bacteria passing out with the faeces are constantly being replenished by multiplication of the population in the gut lumen.

In my laboratory attempts have been made to model the rat hindgut ecosystem using a continuous culture system or chemostat (7,8). Others have utilized semi-continuous culture, in which the growth medium is added as discrete batches (usually twice a day), to model the human gut ecosystem (9).

2. <u>PROCEDURES</u>

<u>Simulation of the rat intestinal ecosystem</u>

In determining the similarity between the <u>in vitro</u> model system and the mammalian gut, the following criteria are likely to be important and are considered in the present paper:

a. relative proportions of the major groups of organisms

b. community structure of the bacterial population in terms of major genera and species

c. metabolic activity and enzymic complement.

<u>Proportions of the major groups of organisms</u>. In our initial studies, freshly collected faeces from a Wistar or Sprague-Dawley rat were used to inoculate the growth medium, based on Oxoid

Reinforced Clostridial Medium (7) in a type 500 modular fermenter
(L.H. Engineering). The cultures (600 ml final volume) were
maintained at 37° under an anaerobic atmosphere and agitated at
300 rpm.

Although various combinations of pH and dilution rate of culture
were tried, it was not possible to retain all of the major groups of
intestinal organisms in culture (7). Thus, in order to provide
favourable environmental conditions for all groups (low pH for
lactobacilli, more neutral pH for anaerobes and enterobacteria) an
in vitro system with differential culture conditions was devised,
comprising two culture vessels connected in series, so that the
output from the first vessel became the input for the second vessel
(Fig.1).

FIGURE 1. Diagram of two-stage continuous culture system

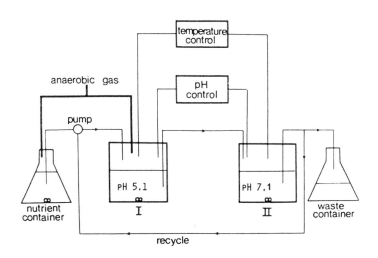

A further refinement was the inclusion of a cell recycle in
which culture medium from stage II was recycled to stage I at one
tenth the rate of flow of fresh medium. This effectively extends

the retention time of species in the culture system and markedly
improves the species diversity of the final population (7). Using
such a system with stages I and II poised at pH 5.1 and 7.1
respectively, a population of organisms developed which closely
resembled the rat faecal flora on the basis of bacterial group
proportions (Table 1). It should be noted that the faecal and
caecal bacterial populations of the rat are very similar (Rowland
unpublished observations) but for this study comparisons were made
to the faecal flora since this could be sampled on multiple
occasions from the same animal to obtain data on day to day
variation.

TABLE 1   Comparison of bacterial group proportions in
           Sprague-Dawley rat faeces and in two-stage continuous
           culture.

Bacterial Group	% Total population $\pm$ SEM		
	Faeces	In vitro*	
		Stage I (pH 5.1)	Stage II (pH 7.1)
Anaerobes	81 $\pm$ 10	83 $\pm$ 1	94 $\pm$ 4
Lactobacilli	11 $\pm$ 7	10 $\pm$ 3	3 $\pm$ 1
Streptococci	7 $\pm$ 4	7 $\pm$ 3	2 $\pm$ 1
Enterobacteria	0.8 $\pm$ 0.3	0.5 $\pm$ 0.1	1 $\pm$ 0.5
Staphylococci	0.0006 $\pm$ 0.0006	ND	ND
Total viable count ($\times$ 10^9/g)	9.5	0.2	1.1

Dilution rate 0.07/h.

ND = not detected

*   The percentage of the total viable count contributed by a
     bacterial group was determined at steady state (after 400 hours
     of culture)

Species composition of the in vivo and in vitro ecosystems.
Although the proportions of the bacterial groups (Table 1) reached
approximately constant values, after 150-250h of two-stage
continuous culture, a defined succession of species within the
groups occurred up to 400 hours of culture. After this time,
however, the structure of the bacterial groups remained constant and
showed marked similarities to the species composition of the rat
faecal microbial population (Table 2).

Influence of source of inoculum on final community structure in
vitro. Sprague-Dawley and Wistar rats differed significantly in the
proportions of the major bacterial groups in faeces. When two-stage
continuous culture systems were inoculated with faeces from the
different rat strains, the community structure of the population
which developed reflected the bacterial group proportions and the
species composition of the rat strain from which the inoculum was
taken (7). This indicates that the hind gut flora is a highly
organised community, with a great capacity for self-regulation and
homeostasis.

Production of short-chain fatty acids. A wide variety of
short-chain fatty acids, similar to those in rat faeces, was
detected in the continuous culture system (Fig. 2). The
concentration of the acids attained an approximate steady state 7-10
days after inoculation (with the exception of hexanoic acid)
indicating that bacterial metabolism and bacterial numbers are
closely linked (8).

TABLE 2   Comparison of the most common microorganisms in Sprague-Dawley
rat faeces and in continuous culture (in vitro)

Bacterial Group	Faeces	In vitro
Enterobacteria	Escherichia coli (74%) Proteus mirabilis (18%) Klebsiella pneumoniae	Escherichia coli (94%) Proteus mirabilis (6%)
Pseudomonads	Pseudomonas aeruginosa	Pseudomonas aeruginosa
Lactobacilli	Lactobacillus plantarum (55%) L.acidophilus (35%) L. brevis (4%) L. lactis L. buchneri L. leichmannii	Lactobacillus plantarum (54%) L.acidophilus (31%) L. brevis (8%) L. viridescens (6%) Lactobacillus sp. (?) L. lactis
Streptococci	Streptococcus salivarius (94%) S. sanguis (5%) S. mitis S. faecalis	Streptococcus salivarius (81%) S. faecalis (15%) S. sanguis (3%) S. bovis S. mitis
Anaerobes	Bacteroides thetaiotaomicron (40%) B. fragilis (30%) B. melaninogenicus Bacteroides spa. (?) B. oralis Bifidobacterium bifidum Peptostreptococcus sp. (?)	Bacteroides thetaiotaomicron (55%) B. melaninogenicus (20%) B. vulgatus (16%) Bifidobacterium spa. (?) (3%) Bacteroides sp[a] (?) Clostridium sp.[a] (?) Bifidobacterium bifidum

The species are listed in order of numerical abundance. Values
in parentheses show the abundance of each species as a percentage of
the totala viable count for that bacterial group; where no values
are given, the species contributed less than 1% of the total group
count. Isolates followed by (?) were tentatively identified.
Organisms unidentified at the species level are distinguished from
other unidentified species at the same genera by alphabetical
superscripts.

Figure 2   Short chain fatty acids (s.c.f.a.) production by the rat
hind gut flora in continuous culture (Stage II)

Ethanoic   ,   propanoic   ,   butanoic   ,   pentanoic   ,

hexanoic   ,   2-methylpropanoic   ,   3-methylbutanoic

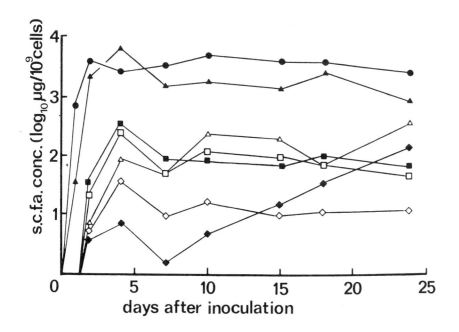

Bacterial enzyme activities

The enzymic activity of the microbial population of stage II was
generally similar, with respect to a range of hydrolytic and
reductive functions, to that of a suspension of fresh caecal
contents (Table 3). However, a major difference was noted in
B-glucuronidase activity which was much more active in caecal
contents than in continuous culture. When the bacterial population
in the chemostat was exposed to a B-glucuronide, B-glucuronidase was
induced and the resulting activity was similar to that in caecal
contents (Table 3). The activities of nitrate reductase and

B-glucosidase could also be induced by their respective substrates indicating that microbial metabolism in the gut may be regulated by exogenous factors such as nitrate and glucosides and by endogenous factors such as glucuronides (products of mammalian hepatic conjugation reactions). Bile acids, in particular cholic acid, were also found to influence some of the enzyme activities, notably B-glucuronidase, B-glucosidase and azoreductase, which were increased, and nitrate reductase, which was decreased (8).

TABLE 3   Comparison of microbial enzyme activities in rat caecal contents and continuous culture. Substrate induction of enzymic activities

Enzyme	umol substrate transformed/h/10" cells		
	Caecal contents	Continuous culture (Stage II)	
		Before Induction*	After Induction*
Azoreductase	3.5 ± 0.3	3.6 ± 0.5	2.9 ± 0.5
Nitroreductase	2.1 ± 0.2	2.5 ± 0.2	2.7 ± 0.2
Nitrate reductase	6.8 ± 0.7	8.4 ± 0.3	10.1 ± 0.3
B-glucosidase	5.9 ± 0.3	7.3 ± 0.6	11.5 ± 0.6
B-glucuronidase	27.3 ± 2.1	4.0 ± 0.2	20.1 ± 0.8

*   The appropriate substrate (0.5 mM final concentration) was added to the culture (Stage II) at zero time ("before induction") and enzyme activities determined after 4 hours ("after induction"). Values shown are means ± SEM (n=4).

It would appear that the products of the enzymic reactions may be similar in the chemostat to those produced in vivo. Thin layer chromatography of the metabolites from the azo dye Brown HT revealed that the continuous culture generated identical metabolites to those

found in faeces of rats exposed to the compound orally. In contrast
batch culture incubations of Brown HT with rat caecal contents gave
a very different metabolic profile.

Semi-continuous culture of human intestinal bacteria

Miller and Wolin (9) have described a semicontinuous culture of
the microbial community of the human large intestine. The system
consisted of 500 ml of nutrient suspension inoculated with human
faeces, to which was added 200 ml of fresh nutrient suspension once
or twice daily, after removal of a similar volume of culture. The
suspension contained sodium deoxycholate, urea, casein, vitamins,
salts and comminuted fibrous foods (lettuce, carrots, celery,
apple-sauce) as the primary carbon-energy source. On the basis of
the rate of volatile fatty acid production, the culture system
resulted in an apparently steady state by 29 days. Acetate was the
major fatty acid product, with butyrate, formate and propionate
being formed in smaller quantities. The gas products of the in
vitro system were similar to those formed in vivo, with both methane
and hydrogen being produced.

The microbial population (about 2×10^9 organisms/g culture)
in the culture system consisted predominantly of anaerobes which
outnumbered the coliforms by about 100:1. Species of Bacteroides,
Fusobacterium, Ruminococcus and Clostridium were isolated from the
culture and these have been shown to be present in large numbers in
human faeces.

On the basis of these bacteriological and fermentation studies,
the semi-continuous culture system would appear to be a good model
of the human large intestinal ecosystem and in particular could
prove extremely useful for studying microbial fermentation and other
microbial activities in the large intestine.

Advantages and uses of continuous culture of gut populations

The continuous and semi-continuous culture systems described
here enable a stable microbial community, closely resembling that in
the mammalian hind gut, to be maintained in vitro for long periods
dissociated from the influences of the host animal. The systems
will therefore facilitate studies of intestinal bacterial
fermentations, other metabolic activities and microbial interactions
over prolonged periods and will help elucidate the factors which
control these reactions and interactions in the gut.

REFERENCES

1. Gorden HA Pesti L. 1972. The gnotobiotic animal as a tool in
    the study of the host microbiol relationships. Bacteriol. Rev.
    35 390-429.

2. Berg RD 1978. Antagonism among the normal anaerobic bacteria of
    the mouse gastrointestinal tract determined by
    immunofluorescence. Appl. Environ. Microbiol 35 1066-1073.

3. Latham MJ Wolin MJ. 1978. Use of a serum bottle technique to
    study interactions between strict anaerobes in mixed culture.
    In 'Techniques for the Study of Mixed Populations', DW Lovelock
    and R Davies (Eds) 113-124. London Academic Press.

4. Freter R Aranki A. 1973. Patterns of interaction in gnotobiotic
    mice among bacteria of a synthetic 'normal' intestinal flora.
    In: 'Germ-free Research. Biological Effect of Gnotobiotic
    Environments' 429-435. SB Henegan (Ed) London Academic Press.

5. Hobson PN Summers R. 1978. Anaerobic bacteria in mixed
    cultures; ecology of the rumen and sewage digesters. In
    Techniques for the study of Mixed Populations. DW Lovelock and
    R Davies (Eds) 125-141. London Academic Press.

6. Slyter LL Nelson W.O Wolin MJ. 1964. Modifications of a device
    for maintenance of the rumen microbial population in continuous
    culture. Appl. Microbiol. 12, 374-377.

7. Veilleux BG Rowland I. 1981. Simulation of the rat intestinal
    ecosystem using a two-stage continuous culture system. J. Gen.
    Microbiol 123, 103-115.

8. Mallett AK Bearne CA Rowland IR. 1983. Metabolic activity and
    enzyme induction in the rat fecal microflora maintained in
    continuous culture. Appl. Environ. Microbiol 46, (in press).

9. Miller TL Wolin MJ. 1981. Fermentation by the human large
    intestine microbial community in an in vitro semicontinuous
    culture system. Appl. Environ. Microbiol. 42, 400-407.

TISSUE CULTURE SYSTEMS FOR THE EXAMINATION OF BACTERIAL VIRULENCE

L.G. GIUGLIANO, M. BARER, G.F. MANN and B.S. DRASAR

1. INTRODUCTION

The initiation of an infection by bacteria and the subsequent development of the pathology is a very complex process. For simplicity, three aspects will be considered: i) attachment ii) resistance to host factors and iii) toxicity. All of these aspects of the problem can be investigated in cell culture. The study of attachment depends on the development of suitable epithelial cell lines. Resistance to host factors is limited by the availability of professional phagocytic cell lines. Toxins and toxicity of many types of bacteria have been examined in cell culture.

The importance of toxins in the pathogenesis of diseases caused by clostridia has focussed attention on these assays. Examination in tissue culture of the infections caused by bacteroides and other non-sporing anaerobes remains problematical. It is likely that the study of resistance to phagocytosis by macrophage cell lines would prove valuable.

Primary tissue culture systems have been used for many years to examine the cytotoxic activity of filtrates prepared from cultures of Clostridium histolyticum, C. perfringens, C. septicum and C. novyi (1). More recently, established cell lines including Chang liver, HeLa and Detroit 6 have been examined (2).

C. difficile is the toxigenic organism most recently associated with pathological conditions in man. The demonstration of C. difficile cytotoxin in the faeces of patients has provided a fresh impulse to the use of tissue culture for the study of clostridial toxins.

We have used a variety of established cell lines and have examined their sensitivity to the classical toxins and enterotoxin of C. perfringens and to the various factors produced by C. difficile. Cell culture systems can also be used to examine the mode of action of the toxins. The use of drugs inhibiting particular aspects of the cellular response may aid in the elucidation of mechanisms. This approach has been used with the C. difficile toxins (5).

The responses of the cells induced by the bacterial toxins studied are most often assessed by microscopic observation of the morphological changes to the cells and by the measurement of the extent of cell damage caused by the toxins. However, the range of cell cultures can be extended by use of other systems of assessment. Two major benefits can result from changed methodology, (i) an improved quantitation of the effects and (ii) a greater specificity of the qualitative response.

Finter (6) established a method for assessing the relative extent of cell damage in tissue culture based on the use of a vital dye such as neutral red. When added to tissue cultures, more dye is taken up by healthy cells than by damaged cells.

The extent of cell damage can be measured indirectly by the neutral red assay described below. The results obtained with this method must be clearly interpreted. Since this method measures directly the amount of dye uptake by healthy cells, it provides an indirect estimation of the extent of cell damage. The cells which were not able to incorporate the dye may be those cells with altered membrane permeability, but which remain attached to the surface of the plate. However, the same results might be explained by a diminished number of attached cells due to cell detachment and loss during washing or by growth inhibition.

This neutral red assay is only one of a whole range of techniques that can be used. In this paper we illustrate how developments in the methods used to assess cellular responses can improve the data generated by cell culture assays of bacterial toxins.

2. MATERIALS AND METHODS

Growth conditions and toxin production

Stock cultures of the strains of C. perfringens used in the study of the sensitivity of mammalian cell lines to enterotoxin were subcultured to 20 ml of fluid-thioglycollate medium (BBL, Cockeysville, MD, USA), heat-shocked at 75°C for 20 minutes and incubated overnight at 37°C. An inoculum (0.2 ml) from the overnight culture was transferred to freshly-steamed fluid-thioglycollate medium (20 ml) and incubated for 6 h at 37°C. An inoculum, (200 ul) of the 6-h culture, was transferred to 20 ml of modified Duncan and Strong medium (DS/R((7), and incubated at 37°C for 18-20 h. DS/R cultures were centrifuged (3000 g for 20 min) and supernates filtered through membrane filters (pore size 0.22 um; Millipore Corp, Bedford, MA, USA). Portions (0.5 ml) of the filtrates were stored at -70°C.

Toxic filtrates of C. difficile were prepared by growing the strains in cooked meat medium for 5 days at 37°C. Cultures were then centrifuged and filtered through a 0.22 um membrane (Millipore Corp).

Cell culture

Ten established mammalian cell lines were used: Chinese
hamster ovary (CHO-K1), mouse adrenal-cortex tumour (Y-1), mouse
areolar and adipose tissue (L-929), African green monkey kidney
(Vero), adult Rhesus monkey kidney (LLC-MK$_2$), rabbit kidney
(RK-13), dog kidney epithelial cells (MDCK), embryonic human
intestine (INT-407), human embryonic foreskin (HFS) and human
embryonic lung (MRC-5).

Y-1 and CHO-K1 cells were grown in Ham Nutrient Mixture F-12
(Flow Laboratories Ltd, Irvine, Ayrshire KA12 8NB, Scotland); Vero
and LLC-MK$_2$ cells in medium 199 with Earle's salts (Flow
Laboratories); MRC-5, HFS, RK-13, MDCK, L-929 and INT-407 cells in
Minimum Essential Medium with Earle's salts (Gibco Europe Ltd). All
media were supplemented with foetal-calf serum (Gibco) 10% v/v,
penicillin G 100 units/ml and streptomycin 100 ug/ml (Glaxo
Laboratories Ltd).

Toxin assays

Serial two-fold dilutions of toxin were prepared in 50 ul
volumes in the wells of microtitre plates (Falcon Microtest II,
Becton Dickinson, USA). Cell suspension was then added in 50 ul
volumes to give 2.5×10^4 cells and a total volume of 100 ul per
well. Negative control wells received diluent and cells only.
Plates were then sealed with self-adhesive film and incubated at
37°C. After 24 hours incubation, the plates were examined
microscopically and toxin titre assessed as the highest dilution of
the preparation showing significant cytological changes relative to
the control wells. Thereafter, medium was discarded from the plates
and 1:10,000 neutral red in 199 medium at pH 7.0 added at 100 ul per
well. After incubation for three hours, neutral red medium was
discarded and wells washed with saline to remove excess dye. Cell

associated dye was extracted by the addition of 100 ul per well of
acidified methanol. Dye concentration was determined at a
wavelength of 492 nm in an automated plate reader
(Titertek-Multiscan). Statistical analyses were performed by probit
linear regression analysis (8).

Antitoxin assays

Serial two-fold dilutions of serum were prepared in 50 ul
volumes in mitrotitre plates. Diluted toxin was then added at 50 ul
per well and the mixture incubated for 1 hour at room temperature.
Vero cell suspension was then added to give a final volume of 150 ul
and 25,000 cells per well. Negative controls consisted of serum
dilutions plus diluent and cells, while positive controls were
diluent plus dilute toxin and cells. In addition, the challenge
dose of toxin was assayed as described above. Plates were then
incubated at 37°C for 24 hours and read as above. Antitoxin titre
was read microscopically as the highest dilution of serum showing a
significant protective effect relative to the positive controls.

Toxin assay (Fig. 1)

Positive control = 154, Negative control = 325,
Difference = 171

Log_{10} dilution	2.6	2.9	3.2	3.5	3.8	4.1
OD 492	157	165	204	253	290	321
% Toxicity	98	94	71	42	20	2.2
Probit	(7.05)	6.55	5.55	4.8	4.16	(2.98)

$$n = 4$$
$$K = 02.64$$

Linear regression $r = 0.995$

$$S = 3.45 = 1:2,821$$

Antitoxin assay

Positive control = 118, Negative control = 281,
Difference = 163

Log$_{10}$ dilution	2.9	3.2	3.5	3.8	4.1
OD 492	274	250	191	132	119
% Toxicity	96	81	45	8.6	0.6
Probit	(6.75)	5.88	4.87	3.63	(2.49

$$n = 3$$
$$K = -3.75$$
Linear regression $\quad r = 0.998$
$$S = 3.44 = 1{:}2{,}785$$

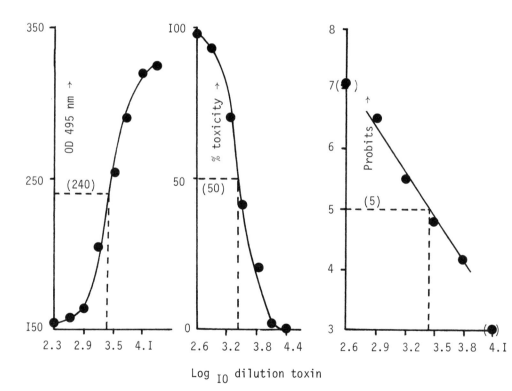

Log $_{10}$ dilution toxin

Figure 1 Qualitative aspects of neutral red assay of
C. difficile cytotoxin on Vero cells

3.   RESULTS

Quantitative aspects of neutral red assay

An example of the results obtained when using neutral red
uptake to assay the cytotoxicity of C. difficile cytotoxin is
presented in Figure 1. The level of effect that can be detected
using this assay is some 8 to 16 times less than that detected by
microscopic examination of the cells. The antitoxin assay is 4-8
times less sensitive in this system. However, the precision of the
assay is much greater. Further the results of the assay in the form
of the slopes of the graphs are characteristic of the toxin examined
but become steeper if the incubation time is extended.

Qualitative aspect of neutral assay
The effect of C. difficile toxin on MRC-5 cells

The morphological effect observed in and the damage to the
MRC-5 cells induced by the filtrates of C. difficile were studied.
It was shown that, when filtrates affected 100% of the cells
morphologically, the percentage of cells damaged varied between 50%
and 68%. However, when the percentage of cells morphologically
affected was 25% or less, the amount of cell damage varied from 18%
to 40%. Figure 2 presents an example of the relationship between
the morphological effect and the cellular damage, as determined by
neutral red assay.

Furthermore, it was noticed that when the filtrates were
dialysed overnight against PBS-A buffer pH 7.0, the inhtensity of
the morphologic effect did not change. However, the percentage of
cells damaged decreased.

Study of the effects of the filtrates of <u>C. difficile</u> treated
with <u>C. sordellii</u> antiserum by the neutral red assay showed that
cell damage still occurred despite the morphological effect being
completely neutralised. Dialysed filtrates treated with
<u>C. sordellii</u> antiserum induced very little cellular damage.

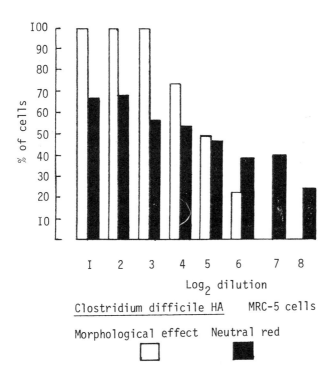

Figure 2 Morphological and neutral red assessment of
C. difficile cytotoxin

Alkali treatment of the filtrate of the strain HA completely
abolished the morphological changes and cellular damage induced by
the filtrates on MRC-5 cells (Figure 3). However, the same
treatment of the filtrate of the strain B, which presented higher
cytotoxic activity than HA, was not completely abolished.

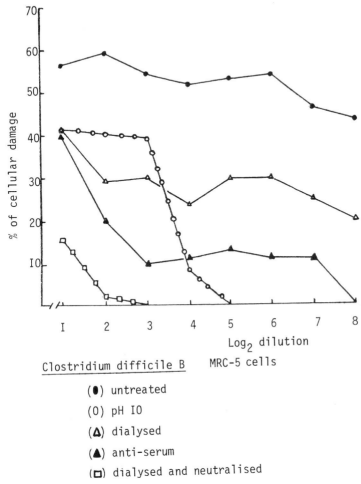

Clostridium difficile B   MRC-5 cells

(●) untreated
(O) pH IO
(△) dialysed
(▲) anti-serum
(□) dialysed and neutralised

Figure 3   Neutral red assay of C. difficile filtrates after
various treatments

Damage caused by the filtrates of C. perfringens type A on Vero cells

Neutral red assays were performed to compare the extent of
damage caused by the enterotoxic filtrates and the morphological
effect observed on Vero cells. It was determined that when all the

198

cells observed were morphologically affected the percentage of cells
damaged varied between 45 and 60%, suggesting that morphological
changes do not necessarily lead to an immediate damage of the
cells. However, when the morphological effect decreased the amount
of cell damage did not decrease in proportion. These results
reinforce the observation that detachment of cells is caused by the
filtrates. Thus, the higher percentage of cell damage, in relation
to the cells morphologically affected could represent the cells
detached from the wells. Figure 4 shows a typical response of the
cells, when inoculated with filtrates, of a strain of
enterotoxigenic C. perfringens.

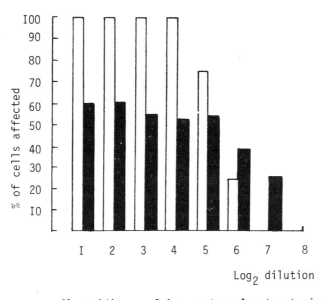

Clostridium perfringens type A enterotoxin

Vero cells
Morphological effect   Neutral red

Figure 4   Morphological and neutral red assessment of
C. perfringens enterotoxin

4. DISCUSSION

The studies reported here illustrate the value of tissue culture systems for the detection and assay of bacterial toxins. Cells are usually assessed morphologically but the studies on the neutral red assay illustrate the potential of other systems of assessment to improve the precision of the assay (Figure 1) and also increase the range of effects that can be detected (Figures 2 and 4). A further extension of this approach would be the use of histochemical stains to examine particular reactions occurring within cells.

A useful result of these studies may be an assay for C. difficile enterotoxin (Figure 3). The treatment of the filtrates with alkali, in an attempt to destroy the cytotoxin and determine the effects of the enterotoxin on the cells was not conclusive, since the filtrates of the different strains tested behaved differently. However, if we assume the alkali treatment to have been effective, the results may be explained by the suggestion that not all strains are equally able to produce enterotoxin. Thus, the effects of strain HA were completely abolished by alkali treatment and dialysis, while filtrates prepared from strain B exhibited a residual activity due to the enterotoxin.

REFERENCES

1. Barg GS. 1937. Action des toxins du groupe de la gangrene ganzense sur les cultures de tissus. Ann. Inst. Pasteur. 59, 536-548.

2. Solotovsky M and Johnson W. 1970. Tissue culture and bacterial protein toxins. Microbial Toxins I, 277-327, London, Academic Press.

3. Giugliano LG Mann, GF and Drasar BS. 1982. Other enterotoxic enteropathies, the use of tissue culture for the detection of clostridial toxins. Europ. J. Chemotherapy and Antibiot, 2, 139-142.

4. Giugliano LG Stringer MF and Drasar BS. 1982. Detection of
    Clostridium perfringens enterotoxin by tissue culture and
    double-gel diffusion methods. J. Med. Microbiol. 16, 233-237.

5. Giugliano LG and Drasar BS. 1983. The influence of drugs on
    the response of a cell culture preparation to bacterial
    toxins. J. Med. Microbiol. (in press).

6. Finter NB. 1969. Dye uptake methods for assessing viral
    cytopathogenicity and their application to interferon assay.
    J. Gen. Virol. 5, 419-427.

7. Labbe RG and Rey DK 1979. Raffinose increases sporulation and
    enterotoxin production by Clostridium perfringens type A.
    Appl. Environ. Microbiol. 37, 1196-1200.

8. Finney DJ. 1954. Statistical method in Biological Assay.
    London, Griffin.

ADHERENCE IN ANAEROBES: AN IN VITRO MODEL OF ADHESION IN
CLOSTRIDIUM DIFFICILE

M.R. BARER

INTRODUCTION

Precendents for the contribution made by adhesion to
pathogenicity are abundant in the study of aerobic bacteria.
Examples include Streptococcus pyogenes and Bordetella pertussis in
the upper respiratory tract, Escherichia coli and Vibrio cholerae in
the small intestine, Salmonella spp and Shigella spp in the large
intestine, and Neisseria gonorrhoeae in the urogenital tract (1,2).
In contrast evidence for the role of adherence in anaerobic
infections is largely circumstantial and, while limited studies have
been performed in animal models (3) and on dental plaque (4), little
is known of the mechanisms involved. The purpose of this work has
been the establishment of an in vitro model for the study of
adherence in obligate anaerobes.

Two forms of evidence can be obtained from studies of adhesion
in vitro. With the first, adhesion is seen as a phenotypic
attribute whose measurement can be correlated with pathogenicity.
The contribution made by the measured phenomenon in vivo need not be
considered. With the second an attempt is made to establish
analogies between events in vitro and the disease process itself.

The now well characterised relationship between the E. coli K88
antigen and piglet diarrhoea serves as a clear example. In this
instance the phenotype detected in vitro, mannose resistant
haemagglutination mediated by the K88 pilus antigen, is plasmid
encoded. Loss of the plasmid is absolutely correlated with loss of
pathogenicity (5). Evidence that elements of the system detected
in vitro are pertinent in vivo is provided by the protective
capacity of antibody to K88 (6). In addition the importance of host

factors in adhesion is highlighted by the discovery that a group of genetically defined disease-resistant piglets exist in whom K88 positive E. coli failed to adhere to intestinal tissue (7).

Sources of evidence for adherence. Table 1 lists the levels at which evidence has been obtained for adhesion as a phenotypic attribute of aerobic bacteria. At the outset when adapting existing methods for use with anaerobes the main problem would appear to be the simultaneous preservation of viability of substrate and bacteria.

Table 1   Levels of evidence for adhesion

1. In vivo associations
   a) Circumstantial: Close associations between pathogen and tissue demonstrated in biopsy or necropsy material which resist disruption.
   b) Experimental: Animal models, e.g. isolated intestinal loop.
2. In vitro models - viable substrate
   a) Exercised tissue: Biopsy or necropsy material e.g. small intestine.
   b) Isolated cell systems: Enterocytes, buccal epithelial cells, eryuthrocytes.
   c) Tissue culture monolayers.
3. In vitro models - non viable substrate
   a) Subcellular fractions: Brush border.
   b) Synthetic substrates: Hydrophobic gels.

In early experiments this was an overriding concern. Studies using non-viable substrates such as brush border preprations, however, illustrate that viability may not be important (8). The work presented reflects this gradual realisation on my part and the consequent selection of methods.

Why study Clostridium difficile? C. difficile, as described elsewhere in this symposium, is the enteropathogen considered responsible for pseudomembranous colitis in man and haemorrhagic caecitis in hamsters. It was selected for study here because he principal virulence factors described to date (toxin A and toxin B) (9) do not fully explain the observed pattern of disease. The role of adhesion in other enterotoxic enteropathies, the initial focal pattern of pathology seen in pseudomembranous colitis, the high carriage rates seen in infants as compared with adults (10) and the existence of a toxin-positive human isolate which is non-pathogenic in hamsters (S P Borriello, personal communication) all suggest that adhesion might be a fruitful area of investigation. In addition, intimate association between C. difficile and colonic mucosa in both human biopsy material and the rat caecum (11, 12) constitutes circumstantial evidence for the contribution of adhesion to pathogenicity.

In most instances the studies described were performed in parallel with an enterotoxigenic strain of Clostridium perfringens type A and a strain of Shigella sonnei. The former was included for interest while the latter was considered a positive control for adhesion to human colonic mucosa.

MATERIALS AND METHODS

Bacterial strains: Clinical isolates of C. difficile from cases of pseudo-membranous colitis and antibiotic-associated colitis were kindly provided by Mr. D. Felmingham (University College Hospital, London). Storage, prior to examination, had been for up to one year in Robertson's cooked meat medium (Southern Group Laboratories). The strains of enterotoxigenic C. perfringens and Shigella sonnei were drawn from laboratory stock and had originally been isolated from individuals with diarrhoea.

Growth conditions: In all experiments inocula were prepared by touching five well separated colonies on solid media and inoculating either C. difficile agar (Oxoid Ltd) supplemented with 7% horse blood (without antibiotic supplement) or fluid thioglycollate medium (Oxoid Ltd). After 48 hours growth at 37°C under anaerobic conditions test suspensions were prepared by washing colonies from the surface of solid medium or from broth culture by centrifugation. These were washed twice in phosphate buffered

204

saline pH 7.2 (PBS) and resuspending in test medium. Various test
media were tried in all procedures described below. In principle
they constituted an environment favourable to either clostridia or
cell substrate. The former included thioglycollate broth, PBS +
0.03% sodium formaldehyde sulphoxylate, PBS + 0.5% cysteine, VPI
dilution salts, and the latter included unsupplemented PBS and cell
culture medium.

Test systems evaluated. Segments of resected human colon,
appearing normal to naked eye inspection, were obtained from
colectomy specimens (by kind permission of Professior C G Clark,
University College Hospital).

All resections had been performed for colonic carcinoma. The tissue
was transported to the laboratory within one hour of resectioin and
was maintained in minimal essential medium (MEM) (Gibco Ltd) + 1%
foetal calf serum (FCS) containing pencillin 100 U/ml and
Streptomycin 100 ug/ml. The tissue was washed twice in sterile PBS
prior to exposure.

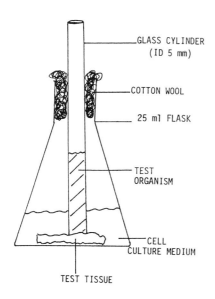

GLASS CYLINDER
(ID 5 mm)

COTTON WOOL

25 ml FLASK

TEST
ORGANISM

CELL
CULTURE MEDIUM

TEST TISSUE

The apparatus shown in Figure 1
was used in all experiments.
Washed 1 cm square segments of
tissue were dropped into the
conical flask (containing 10 ml
MEM + 1% FCS without antibiotics)
and secured, mucosal surface
upward, using the glass cylinder
held firmly in place by the cotton
wool bung.

Figure 1

Excess cell culture medium trapped within the cylinder was pipetted off and bacterial suspensions could then be added containing a suitable reducing agent. Initially phosphate buffered saline containing sodium formaldehyde sulphoxylate (0.03%) was used. However it was found that extensive mucosal disruption took place with this agent and subsequently L cysteine (0.5%) was used. After an incubation period of 45 minutes at 37°C the bacterial suspension was pipetted off and the exposed mucosal surface was washed gently, once, in PBS. The glass cylinder and cell culture medium were then removed and the whole tissue fragment washed twice in 10 ml PBS. Attached bacteria were then 'released' by stomaching the washed tissue for 30 mins in 3 ml releasing fluid. Initially this consisted of 1% SDS in PBS with added sodium formaldehyde sulphoxylate. However, SDS was found to be toxic to C. difficile and subsequently PBS alone was used. Viable bacteria released by the procedure were counted after serial tenfold dilutions, on using a modified Miles and Misra technique, C. difficile agar (Oxoid Ltd) with added selective supplement.

Buccal epithelial cells. The method of Candy et al (13) was used in all its essential elements. Buccal epithelial cells (BEC) were obtained by scraping one end of a clean glass slide along the inside of the author's buccal mucosa (twice on each side) and washing the cells off with 5 ml sterile PBS. Cells were washed twice in PBS and harvested by centrifugation (700 g for 5 mins and resuspended to a concentration of approximately 10^{5} cells/ml). 0.2 ml of this suspension was then mixed with 0.2 ml of bacterial suspension, prepared as described above, in an Eppendorf tube. Mixtures were incubated horizontally with shaking (200 rpm) at 37°C for 45 minutes. The suspension was then washed five times in PBS by centrifugation at 700 g for 30 secs. The resulting pellet was resuspended in 50 ul PBS, smeared on a glass slide, air dried, heat fixed and Gram stained. Adherent bacteria were then enumerated by counting numbers of Gram positive rods per cell and percentage cells with adherent bacteria (100 cells examined).

Intestine 407 cells in suspension. The procedure described above for BEC was conducted with suspensions of intestine 407 cells prepared by treatment of confluent monolayers with trypsin/EDTA and resuspension in MEM + 10% FCS. Suspensions were allowed 1 hour to 'recover' from trypsinisation prior to washing in PBS and proceeding as described. Suspensions were prepared at 10^6 cells/ml.

Intestine 407 cell monolayers. Cells were grown to confluency in MEM + 10% FCS and antibiotics on the surface of sterile circular glass or plastic cover slips placed in the wells of 24 well plastic tissue culture trays (Falcon Plastics Ltd). Prior to exposure the monolayers were washed once with sterile PBS. Bacterial suspensions were added to the wells and incubated for varying periods of time at $37^\circ C$. At the end of exposure, bacterial suspensions were pipetted off, the monolayers washed firmly three times with PBS, fixed in 10% buffered formaldehyde and Gram stained. Adhesion was assessed by examining 300 cells per preparation and enumerating percentage cells with adherent bacteria and mean number of bacteria per cell.

RESULTS

Resected human colon. In the twenty strains examined no evidence for adhesion could be found. Parallel studies performed with the laboratory strain of Shigella sonnei consistently gave viable counts of approximately 10^6 bacteria per cm^2 of exposed mucosa.

Buccal epithelial cells. Gram positive rods were found consistently in association with BEC. However only in very occational preparations did bacteria appear to be significantly more associated with cells than supernatant. Experiments were originally performed using suspensions containing reducing agents. After it was discovered that this made no significant difference to bacterial viability over the incubation period used (45 mins), suspensions were made in PBS without reducing agents. In contrast, significant numbers of cell associated bacteria were found in experiments with S. sonnei.

Intestine 407 cells in suspension

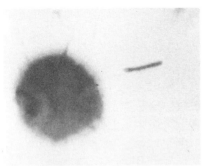

Results were similar to those seen with BEC with very few preparations (including those made with S. sonnei) showing significant cell association. Despite this all clostridial preparations contained the striking morphological associations shown in Figure 2. It was this observation that stimulated the preparation of monolayers with 'adherent' bacteria for the purpose of obtaining scanning electron micrographs of these associations.

Figure 2 Gram stain of INT 407 cell with 'adherent' bacterium

Intestine 407 cell monolayers. Preliminary results suggest that it will be possible to make a systematic appraisal of adhesion in C. difficile using this procedure. The results of an experiment to determine the influence of incubation time on levels of adhesion are presented in Figure 3. It will be noted that levels of adhesion obtained in all three strains rise sharply between 90 and 180 minutes and that levels of adherence are consistently higher in S. sonnei than in both clostridial species examined. Other experiemtns which require further confirmation suggest that adhesion may be enhanced by the presence of cytotoxin-containing culture filtrates and that it may be important for the cell substrate to be viable, while the state of clostridial viability is not relevant. Supporting this latter contention Figures 4 and 5 show scanning electron micrographs of intestine 407 cells with adherent C. difficile. In particular, the appearance in Figure 5 is suggestive of an active process on behalf of the cell substrate. Interestingly in parallel experiments performed with C. perfringens this appearance has not been evident.

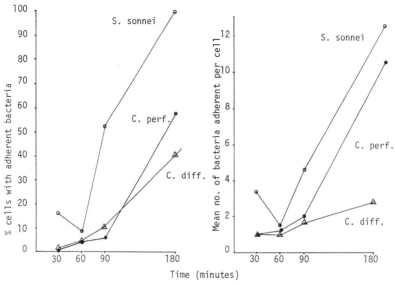

Time (minutes)

Figure 3 Adhesion to INT 407 monolayers. Bacterial suspensions in MEM cell culture medium. C. difficile, C. perfringens, S. sonnei. Mean values from 2-5 preparations are presented.

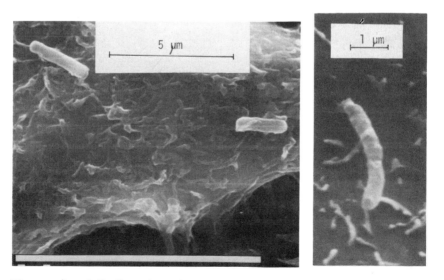

Figures 4 and 5 Scanning electron micrographs of C. difficile adherent to INT 407 monolayers.

DISCUSSION

Methods. The relative amounts of useful data generated with
the four procedures used may, at least in part, reflect problems of
sensitivity and exposure time. The minimum level at which adhesion
could be detected, using the resected colon system, can be
calculated as follows:

Minimum viable count detectable in this system (2 colonies per
33 ul drop) = 60 cfu/ml hence maximum number of adherent cells
detectable (3 ml releasing fluid) = 3 x 60 = 180 cfu/ml.

Assuming similar levels of adherence in Intestine 407
monolayers and colonic enterocytes after 45 minutes incubation,
4% of enterocytes will have 1 adherent bacterium (values from
Figure 2). Total surface area of mucosa exposed

$$= \text{x (internal radius of glass cylinder (um))}^2$$
$$= \text{x } (2.5 \times 10^3) = 19.6 \times 10^6 \text{ um}^2$$

If enterocytes present a surface area of 30 x 30 um then the
estimated number of exposed enterocytes

$$= \frac{19.6 \times 106}{30 \times 30} = 2.18 \times 104$$

Hence maximum number of expected adherent bacteria

$$= 4\% \text{ of } 2.18 \times 10^4 = 872$$

It is not difficult to imagine that aspects of the procedure
itself (failure of bacteria to release during stomaching, and loss
of viability) could account for a fourfold drop in sensitivity,
thereby rendering the procedure unable to detect adhesion. A
similar calculation performed on data from S. sonnei suggests an
expected viable count of 5×10^4 cfu cm^{-2} comparing favourably
with 10^6 cfu cm^{-2} quoted earlier.

Similarly it can be appreciated that if washing fails to eliminate completely bacteria from the supernatant in experiments with BEC and intestine 407 cells in suspension, the level of sensitivity of the assay is set by the number of bacteria per unit area of smear. Thus, if there are 10 bacteria per high power field in cell free areas of the smear and each cell presents an approximate surface area of one fifth of a high power field then the level of adhesion required for detection must exceed 2 bacteria per cell. The results obtained with intestine 407 monolayers suggest that, over the 45 minute incubation period used this is unlikely to be the case.

It seems likely that, were the incubation times used in the cell suspension systems and the resected colon extended, useful data could be obtained. It would be particularly attractive to confirm this with BEC, since a comparison between infant and adult BEC could then be possible.

Results. Preliminary data have been presented here which are consistent with the hypothesis that an association which resists disruption by washing is formed under aerobic conditions between C. difficile and monolayers of intestine 407 cells. The scanning electron microscope (SEM) studies and preliminary LM studies suggest that cell viability may be more important than clostridial viability in this association. Similar structures to those observed by SEM here, have been reported previously with enterobacteriacaeae adherent to cultured monolayers (14). Bacteria were thought to be embedded in glycocalyx material around which the finger-like cellular processes extended. The suggested involvement of active cellular processes in mucosal invasion by Salmonella typhimurium (15) raises the possibility that these structures represent an early stage of cellular invasion.

The relevance of these findings to the possible situation pertaining in vivo cannot be assessed at this stage, particularly since the experiments were conducted under aerobic conditions. Clearly the intestine 407 monolayer system presents a promising prospect for the investigation of adherence phenomena in C. difficile.

References

1. Berkely RCW, Lynch JM, Melling J, Rutter PR, Vincent B. (Eds) 1980. Microbial Adhesion to Surfaces. Ellis Horwood Ltd.
2. Elliott K, O'Connor M, Whelan J. 1981. Adhesion and microorganism pathogenicity. Ciba Foundation.
3. Onderdonk AB, Moon ME, Kasper DL and Bartlett JG. 1978. Adherence of Bacteroides Fragilis in vivo. Infection and Immunity 19, 1083-1087.
4. Gibbons RJ. 1980. Adhesion of bacteria to surfaces of the mouth. Microbial Adhesion to Surfaces. Ellis Horewood Ltd.
5. Smith HW, Linggood MA. 1971. Observations on the pathogenic properties of the K88, Hly and Ent plasmids of Escherichia coli with particular reference to porcine diarrhoea. J Med Micro 4: 467-485.
6. Rutter JM, Jones GW. 1973. Protection against enteric disease caused by Escherichia coli - a model for vaccination with a virulence determinant? Nature (Lond) 242: 531-532.
7. Rutter JM, Burrows MR, Sellwood R, Gibbons RA. 1975. A genetic basis for resistance to disease caused by E. coli. Nature (Lond) 257, 135-136.
8. Sellwood R, Gibbons RA, Jones GW, Rutter JM. 1975. Adhesion of enteropathogenic Escherichia coli to pig intestinal brush borders: the existence of two pig phenotypes. J Med Micro 8: 405-411.
9. Sullivan NM, Pellett S, Wilkins TD. 1982. Purification and characterization of toxins A and B of Clostridium difficile: Infection and Immunity 35: 1082-1040
10. Viscide R, Willey S, Bartlett JG. 1981. Isolation rates and toxigenic potential of Clostridium difficile isolates from various patient populations. Gastroenterology 81: 5-9.
11. Borriello SP. 1979. Clostridium difficile and its toxins in the gastrointestinal tract in health and disease. Research and Clinical Forums 1: 33-35.
12. Borriello SP. 1983. Clostridium difficile and gut disease; in Microbes and infections of the gut. CS Goodwin (Ed) Blackwell Scientific Publications, pp 327-345, in press.
13. Candy DCA et al. 1978. Adhesion of enterobacteriaceae to buccal epithelial cells. Lancet 2: 1157-1158.
14. Richmond MH. 1981. Adhesion and Microorganism Pathogenicity, pp 47-55, Ciba Foundation.
15. Jones GW, Richardson LA, Vanden Bosch JL. 1980. In: Microbial Adhesion to Surfaces, pp 211-219. Ellis Horewood Ltd.

ADHESION IN CLOSTRIDIA

P.D. WALKER, THE WELLCOME RESEARCH LABORATORIES, LANGLEY COURT, BECKENHAM, KENT BR3 3BS.

Adhesion is an important stage in the establishment of infectious diseases. Following establishment in the host the symptoms of infection are produced by toxins secreted by the organism. Specific adhesive mechanisms enabling bacteria to attach to mucosal surfaces have been investigated in a number of aerobic species. In particular it has been shown in E.coli that specific adhesins present on the cell are responsible for attachment to the intestinal surface. These include the K88, K99, 987P adhesins responsible for attachment in sheep, cattle and pigs (1-8) and colonization factors 1 and 2 in human E.coli infections.

Because of the success in controlling infection due to clostridial organisms by the use of formal toxoids which stimulate antibodies neutralizing the symptoms of infection, there has been little interest in investigations into the mechanisms by which clostridia adhere to the intestinal surface in enteric infections. That adherence is clearly an important factor is illustrated by examining portions of intestine from piglets and humans infected with C.perfringens type C using the scanning electron microscope. The site of infection is the jejunal villi, shown in Figure 1.

214

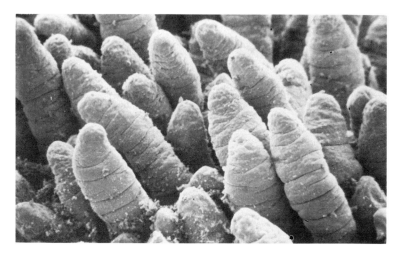

FIGURE 1: Scanning electron micrograph of jejunal villi from a
normal piglet.

Following infection organisms adhere to the intestinal villi
(Figure 2) and as a result of the secretion of toxins necrosis of
the villus surface occurs (Figure 3).

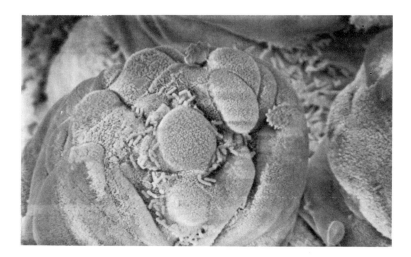

FIGURE 2: Scanning electron micrograph of jejunal villi from
neonatal piglet 4 hours after infection with C.perfringens type C.
Note attachment of the organism to the villus surface.

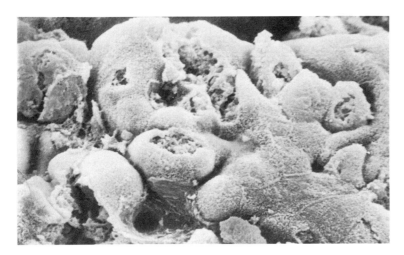

FIGURE 3: Scanning electron micrograph of jejunal villi from a young human adult infected with C.perfringens type C. Note necrosis of villus tips.

In the final stages of infection complete destruction of the villus surface occurs (Figure 4) and organisms can be seen adhering to the necrotic areas (Figure 5).

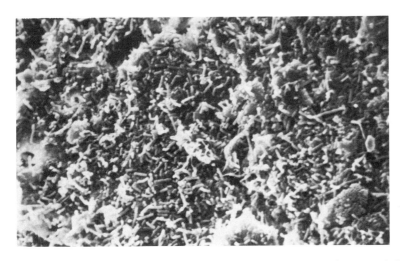

FIGURE 4: Scanning electron micrograph of jejunum from a piglet dying of infection with C.perfringens type C. Note complete destruction of the jejunal villi and adherent organisms.

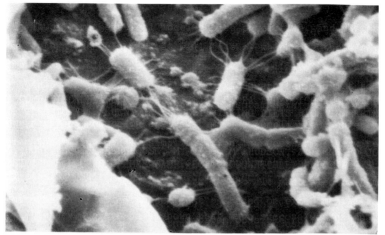

FIGURE 5: Scanning electron micrograph of jejunum from a piglet
dying of infection with C.perfringens type C. Note adherence of
organisms to the surface by fibrous processes.

In the neonatal animal where infection occurs before the
development of a normal bacterial flora, no other organisms are
usually present. In the case of the adult animal the resultant
picture is very complex resulting from the growth and multiplication
of both the pathogen and the normal intestinal flora (Figure 6).

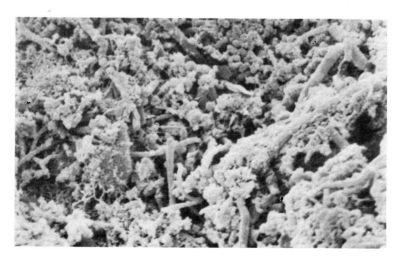

FIGURE 6: Scanning electron micrograph of jejunum of young human
adult infected with C.perfringens type C. Note mixed flora composed
of rods (C.perfringens type C) and coccoid forms.

The picture resembles in many ways the mixed flora seen in similar pictures of plaque in dental caries.

Both proteins and polysaccharide adhesins have been identified as responsible for attachment of bacteria to mucosal surfaces. In the case of clostridia the nature of the attachment is unknown. Recent experience, however, has shown that the study of the mechanisms of attachment may lead to the design of more effective vaccines.

Infections with clostridia occur with either the neonate or adult animal and the presence of circulating antitoxin, produced as a result of vaccination, is normally satisfactory for protection of the animal. In cases where infection is overwhelming due to severe contamination of the external environment, such protection may break down. Infection with C.perfringens type C in piglets is endemic in Denmark (9). The disease originated in localized areas in Jutland and Zeeland but eventually became much more generalized. Protection of the piglets was shown to be correlated with the amount of circulating antitoxin present in the sera, resulting from ingestion of colostrum from the dam (9). In extreme cases, however, even when these required levels of circulating antitoxin are achieved, protection may break down (Hogh, personal communication). It would appear in such circumstances that, in the presence of antitoxin and no significant antiadhesin or bactericidal antibodies, the organism continues to multiply in the intestine and eventually the amounts of toxin produced are such as to overcome the protective antibody.

It has been shown in infections with E.coli that significant protection can be obtained with vaccines containing measured quantities of the specific adhesins (10, 11). Under these

circumstances attachment of the organism to the anterior portion of
the small intestine is prevented and the organism is rapidly
eliminated from the intestine.

There appears to be some evidence in Denmark that protection
with vaccines composed of anacultures (cells plus toxoid) are more
effective than toxoid alone (Hogh, personal communication). If this
is so more effective vaccines could be designed by identifying the
factors responsible for adhesion on the cells and ensuring
sufficient quantities are present in vaccines in combination with
the toxoid.

REFERENCES

1. Isaacson RE, Nagy B and Moon HW. 1977. Colonization of porcine
    small intestine by Escherichia coli; colonization and adhesion
    of piglet enteropathogens that lack K88. Journal of Infectious
    Diseases. 135, 531-538.

2. Orskov I, Orskov F, Smith HW and Sojka WJ. 1975. The
    establishment of K99 a thermolabile transmissible Escherichia
    coli K antigen previously called 'KCO' possessed by calf and lamb
    enteropathogenic strains. Acta Pathologica et Microbiolgica
    Scandinavica Section B, 83, 31-36.

3. Jones GW and Rutter JM. 1972. Role of the K88 antigen in the
    pathogenesis of neonatal diarrhoea caused by Escherichia coli in
    piglets. Infection and Immunity. 6, 918-927.

4. Moon HW, Nagy B, Isaacson RE and Orskov I. 1977. Occurrence of
    K99 antigen on Escherichia coli isolated from pigs and
    colonization of pig ileum by K99+ enterotoxigenic E.coli from
    calves and pigs. Infection and Immunity, 15, 614-620.

5. Nagy B, Moon HW and Isaacson RE. 1976. Colonization of porcine
    small intestine by Eschericia coli: ileal colonization and
    adhesion of pig enteropathogens that lack K88 antigen and by some
    acapsular mutants. Infection and Immunity, 13, 1214-1220.

6. Nagy B, Moon HW and Isaacson RW. 1977. Colonization of porcine
    intestine by enterotoxigenic Escherichia coli: Selection of
    piliated forms in vivo adhesion of piliated forms to epithelial
    cells in vitro and incidence of a pilus antigen among porcine
    enteropathogenic E.coli. Infection and Immunity, 16, 344-352.

7. Smith HW and Linggood MA. 1971. Observations on the pathogenic properties of the K88 and ENT plasmids of Escherichia coli with particular reference to porcine diarrhoea. Journal of Medical Microbiology, 4, 467-485.

8. Smith HW and Linggood MA. 1972. Further observations on Escherichia coli enterotoxins with particular regard to those produced by atypical piglet strains and by calf and lamb strains. The transmissible nature of these enterotoxins and of a K antigen possessed by calf and lamb strains. Journal of Medical Microbiology, 5, 243-250.

9. Hogh P. 1974. Porcin infectious necrotising enteritis caused by Clostridium perfringens. Doctoral Dissertation, Royal Vet.Agr.Univ.Copenhagen.

10. Nagy LK, Walker PD, Bhogal BS and Mackenzie T. 1978. Evaluation of Escherichia coli vaccines against experimental enteric colibacillosis. Res.Vet.Sci. 24, 37-45.

11. Nagy LK and Walker PD. 1983. Multi-adhesin vaccines for the protection of the neonatal piglet against E.coli infections. Develop.Biol.Standard. 53, 189-197.

POSTERS

LIST OF POSTERS

The effect of clavulanic acid on the susceptibility of the B. fragilis group to penicillins.
J.P. Maskell and C.N. Simpson

Antibiotics attenuate experimental hypertension.
J.W. Honour, S.P. Borriello, U. Ganten and P. Honour

Bacteriological and clinical changes during clindamycin induced Clostridium spiroforme-mediated diarrhoea of rabbits.
R.J. Carman and H.B. Waynforth

The demonstration of cross-reactive cell-surface antigen in the genus Clostridium by ELISA
Marie D. Byrne and Ian R. Poxton

Analysis of the LPS antigens of Bacteroides fragilis by western blot transfer.
G. Cousland and Ian R. Poxton

A method for the purification of DNA from poorly-growing anaerobic bacteria and strains with high nuclease activity.
H.N. Shah and R.A. Whiley

Taxonomic studies on some strains previously designated "Bacteroides variabilis" and "Bacteroides incommunis".
H.N. Shah, R. Hammann, R. Brown and M.D. Collins

Production of lignans by colonic bacteria.
S.P. Borriello and K.D.R. Setchell

Colonial variation in Clostridium difficile.
P.N. Levett

Gas chromatography of stools and the detection of Clostridium difficile.
P.N. Levett

Clostridium difficile infection - Protection by prior colonization with non-pathogenic strains.
S.P. Borriello and Fiona Barclay

Colonization resistance of the gastrointestinal tract - A potential in vitro method for the determination of susceptibility to infection with Clostridium difficile.
S.P. Borriello, Fiona Barclay, A.R. Welch

Anaerobiospirillum spp. from animals and man.
H. Malnick, M.E.M. Thomas, H. Lotay and M. Robbins

Motile curved bacilli isolated from the genital tract.
M.S. Sprott, H.R. Ingham, R.S. Pattman, R.L. Eisenstadt, G.R. Short, H.K. Narang, P.R. Sisson, L.M. Clarkson and J.B. Selkon

The pathogenesis of <u>Bacteroides fragilis</u> bacteraemia and tissue
localization in the mouse.
S.C. Baldock, K.G. McCullagh, S. Oswald and A.M.S. Pope

A comparison between the bacterial flora and oligosaccharide content
of ileostomy effluent in subjects taking diets rich in refined or
unrefined carbohydrate.
S. Hori, Louise Barghouse, M. Hill, M. Hudson, J. Lennard-Jones and
Elizabeth Rogers

Influence of dietary lactose and age on the metabolic activity of the
rat caecal microflora.
A.K. Mallett, I.R. Rowland and A. Wise

The effect of diet on the composition of the bacterial flora on the
terminal ileum.
F. Fernandez, H. Kennedy, M. Hill and S. Truelove

Steroid degradation in the gastrointestinal tract - The use of cannulated
pigs as a model system.
K. Fadden, R.W. Owen, M.J. Hill, E. Latymer, G. Low and A.N. Mason

The establishment of complex communities of oral bacteria in the
chemostat using multiple, defined inocula.
Ann S. McDermid, Ailsa S. McKee, P.D. Marsh and D.C. Ellwood

Enhancement of experimental ulcerative colitis by immunization with
<u>Bacteroides vulgatus</u>.
R. Cisneros and A.B. Onderdonk

THE EFFECT OF CLAVULANIC ACID ON THE SUSCEPTIBILITY OF THE
B.FRAGILIS GROUP TO PENICILLINS

J.P. MASKELL AND C.N. SIMPSON. DEPARTMENT OF MEDICAL MICROBIOLOGY,
THE LONDON HOSPITAL MEDICAL COLLEGE, TURNER STREET, LONDON E1 2AD

Fifty recent clinical isolates of the B.fragilis group were
tested to determine their susceptibility to ampicillin,
carbenicillin, mezlocillin, azlocillin and piperacillin using an agar
dilution technique. The influence of clavulanic acid on the
penicillin susceptibility of these strains was determined by
incorporating 2 mg/l of clavulanic acid into test media. The
production of beta-lactamase by the strains was determined by the
nitrocefin test and their isoelectric points by focusing on
polyacrylamide gel. Piperacillin was generally the most active of
the penicillins tested and carbenicillin the least active with
MIC_{50} values of 8 and 32 respectively. Although mezlocillin was
slightly more active than piperacillin against highly resistant
strains (MIC 64 mg/l ampicillin) it was less active against strains
with moderate resistance (16-32 mg/l ampicillin). The majority of
resistant strains became at least fivefold more susceptible to
ampicillin and carbenicillin in the presence of clavulanic acid,
while this effect was less marked for the acylureidopenicillins. In
18% of strains the susceptibility to all five penicillins tested was
virtually unaffected by the presence of clavulanic acid. Of eleven
highly resistant (MIC 64 mg/l) ampicillin isolates obtained from
this and a previous survey, nine showed a substantial reduction in
MIC with all five penicillins in the presence of clavulanic acid.
Three of these strains (two B.fragilis, one B.distasonis) showed up
to an eightfold reduction in MIC with some of the
acylureidopenicillins. The MICs of the remaining two strains (one
B.fragilis, one B.thetaiotaomicron) to the acylureidopenicillins
were virtually unaffected by clavulanic acid.

ANTIBIOTICS ATTENUATE EXPERIMENTAL HYPERTENSION

J.W. HONOUR,[+] S.P. BORRIELLO, U. GANTEN[#] AND P. HONOUR
+ - Cobbold Laboratories, Middlesex Hospital, London W1N 8AA
  - MRC Clinical Research Centre, Harrow HA1 8UJ
- Pharmacology Institute, University Heidelberg D6900 FRG

In rats steroids are largely excreted in bile. Bacteria in the intestine modify the steroids and the products are efficiently reabsorbed into the enterohepatic circulation (EHC). Rats reared germ-free or given certain antibiotics have higher faecal excretion of steroids and faster steroid turnover than normal rats. This study considered the possibility that some of the hypertensive response to steroid hormones is attributable to bacterial metabolites. Over 5 days corticosterone (4 mg/d, IM) raised the blood pressure of Sprague-Dawley rats (n = 6) from 108 to 133 mmHg. For 12 days neomycin (11 mg/kg/d) or vancomycin (20 mg/kg/d) were added to the water of an additional number of rats. Over 7 days the antibiotics alone had no effects on blood pressure but when these rats were additionally challenged with corticosterone for 5 days, the blood pressures increased to 119 and fell to 105 mmHg respectively and were then significantly lower than in response to corticosterone alone. Hypertension was also produced when endogenous steroid secretion was increased by administration of adrenocorticotrophic hormone (Synacthen, 100 ug/d). Blood pressure increased over 5 days from 109 to 151 mmHg in response to ACTH but in rats receiving neomycin, simultaneously, blood pressure rose to 121 mmHg following the ACTH challenge. Neomycin also attenuated the development of high blood pressure in spontaneously hypertensive rats of stroke-prone substrain. These results suggest that experimental hypertension can be modulated by the administration of antibiotics which, presumably, affect the action of gut bacteria in modifying steroids in the EHC.

BACTERIOLOGICAL AND CLINICAL CHANGES DURING CLINDAMYCIN INDUCED
CLOSTRIDIUM SPIROFORME-MEDIATED DIARRHOEA OF RABBITS

R.J. CARMAN AND H.B. WAYNFORTH. ANIMAL UNIT, CHARING CROSS HOSPITAL
MEDICAL SCHOOL, ST.DUNSTAN'S ROAD, LONDON W6 8RP

Caecally fistulated and isolated rabbits were given i.p.
clindamycin and 7 days later 10^5 iota-like toxigenic C.spiroforme
NCTC 11493 per os. Clostridia in caecal samples taken at frequent
intervals were enumerated and iota-like toxin titrated. C.spiroforme
was detected about 7 to 10 hours post challenge (pc), rising to
10^6 cfu/g by 20 hours. The in vivo generation time was as low as
1.3 hours. From 21 hours pc until death the numbers rose to
10^7 cfu/g. C.tertium, C.sporogenes and C.perenne, which were
detectable before challenge, could not be isolated after 20 hours
pc. At no time were C.perfringens, C.difficile, or their toxins,
detected. Iota-like toxin was first detected about 20 hours pc.
Its titre rose from 1 to 64 at death. Caecal fluidity was first
seen at 23 hours. Frank scouring and faecal soiling of the perineum
were observed only 3 to 5 hours before death. Thereafter there were
increasing signs of distress such as apathy, hunched posture,
cyanosis, decreased body temperature, recumbency and hind limb
paralysis. Less frequently the rabbits became convulsive. Although
the time of the onset of clinical and bacteriological signs of
diarrhoea varied, it was unusual for rabbits to survive much beyond
30 hours pc.

Caecal fistulation reveals that experimental C.spiroforme-
mediated diarrhoea is an acute and fatal disease, resembling the
spontaneous condition as closely as can be determined. The
technique can be adapted to investigate further aspects of the
pathogenesis of this and other diseases.

THE DEMONSTRATION OF CROSS-REACTIVE CELL-SURFACE ANTIGEN IN THE
GENUS CLOSTRIDIUM BY ELISA

MARIE D. BYRNE AND IAN R. POXTON, BACTERIOLOGY DEPARTMENT,
UNIVERSITY OF EDINBURGH MEDICAL SCHOOL, EDINBURGH EH8 9AG.

Cell surface antigens were extracted by EDTA from 23 species of
clostridia and reacted in an ELISA with 10 reference whole cell
antisera. The results are summarised below.

EDTA antigen prepared from:	Titre* of reaction between EDTA antigen and antiserum raised against whole cells of the following species:									
	C. perfringens A	C. chauvoei	C. septicum	C. tertium	C. cadaveris	C. sordelli	C. difficile	C. histolyticum	C. sporogenes	C. novyi A
C. perfringens A–E										
C. paraperfringens										
C. absonum										
C. chauvoei										
C. septicum										
C. tertium										
C. fallax										
C. butyricum										
C. perenne										
C. cadaveris										
C. sordelli										
C. bifermentans										
C. difficile										
C. irregularis										
C. histolyticum										
C. sporogenes										
C. novyi A										
C. novyi B										
C. novyi C										
C. novyi D										
C. botulinum A										
C. botulinum pB										
C. botulinum npB										
C. botulinum C										
C. botulinum D										
C. botulinum E										
C. tetani										
C. ramosum										
C. paraputrificum										
C. subterminale										
C. nexile										

* Titre indicated as a fraction of the homologous titre.

●T ●$T/2$ ●$T/4$ ●$T/8$ ●$T/16$ •$T/32$

ANALYSIS OF THE LPS ANTIGENS OF <u>BACTEROIDES FRAGILIS</u> BY WESTERN BLOT
TRANSFER

GARY COUSLAND AND IAN R. POXTON, BACTERIOLOGY DEPARTMENT, UNIVERSITY
OF EDINBURGH MEDICAL SCHOOL, EDINBURGH EH8 9AG.

LPS preparations from 3 strains of <u>B. fragilis</u> were analysed by
sodium dodecyl sulphate-polyacrylamide gel electrophoresis (SDS-PAGE).
The antigenic components of these preparations were then identified by
Western blot transfer and subsequent reaction with anti-<u>B. fragilis</u>
sera.

The SDS-PAGE profiles of LPS from <u>B. fragilis</u> show similarities to
those previously obtained with <u>E. coli</u> and <u>S. typhimurium</u>. The
presence of multiple, regularly-spaced bands has been interpreted in
these species as representing LPS molecules possessing increasing
numbers of side chain repeat units and this is probably also the case
in the present study. The heavily stained LMW* components can be
interpreted as representing rough LPS with a very short saccharide
chain. Most of the HMW* diffuse bands seen in the present study have
not normally been present in SDS-PAGE analyses of enterobacterial LPS
(1), indicating contamination with non-LPS polysaccharide(s).

Western blotting showed that the HMW polysaccharides were
antigenic, but did not represent common antigens. However, 2 LMW
bands, probably corresponding to rough LPS, represented antigens common
to the 3 test strains. The recent suggestion by Kasper <u>et al</u>., (2)
that <u>B. fragilis</u> LPS may contain a common <u>B. fragilis</u> antigen, supports
this finding. However, analysis of LPS antigens from a greater number
of strains is required to confirm that these are true common antigens.

* LMW = low molecular weight;   HMW = high molecular weight.

REFERENCES

1.   Tsai CM and Frasch CE. (1982). Anal.Biochem. <u>119</u>: 115.
2.   Kasper DL, Weintraub A, Lindberg AA and Lonngren J. (1983).
      J.Bacteriol. <u>153</u>: 991.

A METHOD FOR THE PURIFICATION OF DNA FROM POORLY-GROWING ANAEROBIC
BACTERIA AND STRAINS WITH HIGH NUCLEASE ACTIVITY

H.N. SHAH AND R.A. WHILEY. DEPT. OF ORAL MICROBIOLOGY, LONDON
HOSPITAL MEDICAL COLLEGE, TURNER STREET, LONDON E1 2AD.

A procedure has been developed, suitable for the rapid and
routine isolation and purification of DNA from poorly-growing
bacterial species e.g. Bacteroides ureolyticus, or strains producing
nucleases, e.g. B.hypermegas and B.multiacidus. Bacterial cells
were harvested from blood agar plates and treated up to the first
precipitation step of Marmur's method. Two mls. of crude DNA
extract was applied to a column (1.5 x 45 cm) containing Fractogel
65 (B.D.H.), previously equilibrated with SSC. Fractions (1.8 mls)
were collected and the peak heights detected with a 260 nm recorder
(LKB). An optimum combination of column bed height (33 cm) and flow
rate (0.35 ml) min^{-1}) was derived by varying both parameters. DNA
obtained in the first peak fraction was precipitated with ethanol,
re-dissolved in SSC and the mole % G+C estimated by thermal
denaturation. The values obtained for B.fragilis (NCTC 8560) were
42-43%, B.ureolyticus (NCTC 10941) 29-30%, B.hypermegas (3 strains)
32-34% and B.multiacidus (3 strains) 56-58%.

These results are in excellent agreement with published data.
Furthermore the hyperchromicity of DNA prepared by this method was
high (35-38%). The physical properties of Fractogel, for example,
its resistance to compression and organic solvents, make it an ideal
medium for separating large polymers such as DNA.

TAXONOMIC STUDIES ON SOME STRAINS PREVIOUSLY DESIGNATED "BACTEROIDES VARIABILIS" AND "BACTEROIDES INCOMMUNIS"

H.N. SHAH, R. HAMMANN*, R. BROWN AND M.D. COLLINS. DEPT. OF ORAL MICROBIOLOGY, LONDON HOSPITAL MEDICAL COLLEGE, TURNER STREET, LONDON E1 2AD.

The species "Bacteroides variabilis" and "Bacteroides incommunis" are not recognized in the eight edition of Bergey's 'Manual of Determinative Bacteriology' (Buchanan and Gibbons, 1974) nor are they included in the 'Approved Lists of Bacterial Names' (Skerman et al., 1980). In the present study, strains previously designated "B.variabilis" and "B.incommunis", including some fresh isolates, have been examined using biochemical, serological and chemical techniques, in an attempt to clarify their taxonomy. All the strains produced major amounts of succinic and acetic acids, contained malate and glutamate dehydrogenases, predominantly straight chain saturated and methyl branched long chain fatty acids, menaquinones as their sole respiratory quinones (major components, MK-10 and MK-11) and possess a G+C content of ca 40 to 46 mol%. These data, together with the presence of pentose phosphate pathway enzymes (glucose-6-phosphate and 6-phosphogluconate dehydrogenases), indicate that "B.variabilis" and "B.incommunis" most closely resemble the "B.fragilis" group of organisms. Some strains, however, were phenotypically quite distinct from members of the "B.fragilis" group and reacted only with antiserum prepared to strain VPI 11368 ("B.variabilis") using an indirect ELISA technique (Poxton, et al., 1982). These results together with preliminary DNA-DNA reassociation data support the recognition of the species "B.variabilis". Strains presumptively identified as "B.incommunis" were, however, found to be biochemically and serologically indistinguishable from B.vulgatus.

REFERENCE

1. Poxton IR, Brown R & Collee JG. (1982). J.Med.Micro.15, 223.

* Supported by the Deutsche Forschungsgemeinschaft, Bonn (BO 212).

PRODUCTION OF LIGNANS BY COLONIC BACTERIA

S.P. BORRIELLO AND K.D.R. SETCHELL.   CLINICAL RESEARCH CENTRE,
WATFORD ROAD, HARROW, MIDDLESEX HA1 3UJ.

Lignans had only been found in higher plants until the recent
description of enterolactone and enterodiol as the major lignans
present in the urine of humans (1,2). Initial interest in these
compounds was stimulated by the demonstration of a cyclic excretion
pattern during the menstrual cycle, which was suggestive of a
physiological role. Recent work has shown that synthetic
enterolactone is cytotoxic to human lymphoid cells (3) and that it
can significantly depress oestrogen-stimulated rat uterine cytosol
RNA synthesis (4). In addition many lignans are effective against
animal tumours and some have been subjected to clinical trials,
leading to the speculation that they may be involved in a protective
capacity with cancer in man. It has recently been shown that lignan
excretion is lower in women who have breast cancer than in healthy
controls (5). We have shown that excretion of these compounds is
depressed in subjects receiving antibiotics (3). This was
presumptive indirect evidence that the gastrointestinal flora
probably played a part in the production of these compounds in man.
We have now shown that these compounds can be formed _in vitro_ by the
faecal flora and demonstrated that enterolactone is the oxidised
product of enterodiol. This metabolic step is carried out by
facultative bacteria. In addition we have been able to produce both
lignans from linseeds and from secoisolariciresinol, a constituent
of linseed; this reaction is again carried out by facultative
bacteria. Enterolactone has also been produced from matairesinol, a
more abundant plant lignan than secoisolariciresinol, after
incubation under either aerobic or anaerobic conditions. There
appear to be a number of similar operative pathways capable of
producing enterolactone and enterodiol, depending on the major
dietary precursor ingested.

REFERENCES

1. Setchell KDR, Lawson AM, Mitchell FL, et al. 1980. Lignans in man and animal species. Nature, 287: 740-742.

2. Stitch SR, Toumba JK, Groen MB, et al. 1980. Excretion, isolation and structure of a new phenolic constituent of female urine. Nature 287: 738-740.

3. Setchell KDR, Lawson AM, Borriello SP, et al. 1981. Lignan formation in man : microbial involvement and possible roles in relation to cancer. Lancet 2: 4-7.

4. Waters AP and Knowles JT. 1982. Effect of lignan (HPMF) on RNA synthesis in the rat uterus. J.Reprod.Fertil. 66: 379-381.

5. Adlercreutz H, Heikkinen R, Woods M, et al. 1982. Excretion of the lignans enterolactone and enterodiol and of equol in omnivorous and vegetarian post-menopausal women and in women with breast cancer. Lancet 2: 1295-9.

COLONIAL VARIATION IN CLOSTRIDIUM DIFFICILE

P.N. LEVETT. PHLS ANAEROBE REFERENCE UNIT, PUBLIC HEALTH
LABORATORY, LUTON & DUNSTABLE HOSPITAL, LUTON LU4 ODZ

Five isolates of Clostridium difficile have been encountered
which exhibit marked colonial variation. These strains were isolated
from the stools of five patients suffering from antibiotic-associated
diarrhoea; subcultures from primary isolation plates yielded
mixtures of two colony types. Repeated subcultures on horse blood
agar plates yielded pure cultures of both colony types.

One colony type, described as "smooth", produced raised, umbonate
colonies, 2-4 mm across, with irregular margins. The second type,
described as "rough", produced highly irregular colonies with
rhizoidal edges. The two variants did not differ biochemically (see
Table 1). In addition, both types appeared morphologically similar
in Gram-stained films, being Gram-positive bacilli with oval,
sub-terminal spores.

TABLE 1 Biochemical tests for the identification of Clostridium
         difficile

Acid from:	aesculin	maltose	salicin
	arabinose	mannitol	sorbitol
	cellobiose	mannose	starch
	fructose	melezitose	sucrose
	glucose	melibiose	trehalose
	inositol	raffinose	xylose
	lactose	ribose	

Hydrolysis of:	aesculin	Production of:	indole
	gelatin		lecithinase
	starch		lipase
			p-cresol
Reduction of:	nitrate		volatile fatty acids
			(acetic to
			iso-caproic)

However, when negative-stained preparations were examined by transmission electron microscopy, bacteria of the rough colonial type were found to possess numerous peritrichous flagella. In contrast, those of the smooth colonial type were either aflagellate or possessed only a few flagella.

The significance of this observation with regard to the pathogenicity of C.difficile is, as yet, undetermined.

GAS CHROMATOGRAPHY OF STOOLS AND THE DETECTION OF CLOSTRIDIUM
DIFFICILE

P.N. LEVETT. PHLS ANAEROBE REFERENCE UNIT, PUBLIC HEALTH
LABORATORY, LUTON & DUNSTABLE HOSPITAL, LUTON LU4 ODZ

Gas chromatographic detection of iso-caproic acid (IC) has been
recommended as a screening test for the presence of Clostridium
difficile in stools (1). Subsequent work in this laboratory has
produced similar data but our interpretation differs from that of
Potvliege et al. (1).

Sixty stools from patients suspected of having C.difficile -
associated diarrhoea were analysed by gas chromatography for the
presence of volatile fatty acids and phenols, cultured for
C.difficile and tested for cytotoxin.

METHODS

Culture Faecal specimens were subjected to alcohol shock treatment
(2) in addition to direct plating on modified CCFA medium (3).

Cytotoxin assay A suspension of faecal material in phosphate
buffered saline (PBS) containing penicillin (100 ug/ml),
streptomycin (100 ug/ml) and metronidazole (100 ug/ml) was
centrifuged at 2000 g for 20 minutes. Cytotoxicity was assayed on
MRC V tissue culture monolayers; a characteristic cytopathic effect
neutralized by C.sordellii antitoxin was considered positive.

Gas chromatography A 50% suspension of faecal material in 1 ml PBS
(without antibiotics) was extracted and analysed on a Pye Unicam
series 104 chromatograph (3, 4) for p-cresol and for IC.

RESULTS AND DISCUSSION

The number of stools in which C.difficile, or its cytotoxin were detected, was 15. Iso-caproic acid (I.C.) was detected in 7 stools of which 4 contained C.difficile or cytotoxin (see Table) but the organism was not associated with any other volatile fatty acid. Para-cresol was detected in 5/25 stools. Ten of which were C.difficile - positive; no association was noted between C.difficile and the presence of p-cresol.

TABLE   Association between Clostridium difficile and iso-caproic acid in stools

		Clostridium difficile		
		Detected	Not Detected	Total
Iso-caproic	Positive	4	3	7
acid	Negative	11	42	53
		15	45	60

A significant association was observed between the presence of IC and C.difficile (x^2 = 4.366 with 1 degree of freedom). This was expected, since C.difficile is one of only a few organisms which produce IC in vitro. Despite the association of IC with C.difficile the value of this test, as a marker of C.difficile infection, is negligible, since 73% of stools from which C.difficile was isolated did not contain IC. In addition IC was not always present in successive stools from patients shown to have C.difficile and IC initially.

It is concluded that detection of IC and p-cresol in stools are not satisfactory screening tests for C.difficile.

REFERENCES

1. Potvliege C, Labbe M, Yourassowsky E. Gas-liquid chromatography
   as a screening test for <u>Clostridium difficile</u>. Lancet 1981;
   2: 1105.

2. Borriello SP, Honour P. Simplified procedure for the routine
   isolation of <u>Clostridium difficile</u> from faeces. J.Clin.Pathol.
   1981; <u>34</u>: 1124-1127.

3. Phillips KD, Rogers P.A. Rapid detection and presumptive
   identification of <u>Clostridium difficile</u> by p-cresol production
   on a selective medium. J.Clin.Pathol. 1981; <u>34</u>: 642-644.

4. Willis AT, Phillips KD. 1983. Anaerobic Infections. PHLS
   Monograph 3. 2nd ed. London, H.M.S.O.

CLOSTRIDIUM DIFFICILE INFECTION - PROTECTION BY PRIOR COLONIZATION WITH NON-PATHOGENIC STRAINS

S.P. BORRIELLO AND FIONA BARCLAY.   CLINICAL RESEARCH CENTRE, WATFORD ROAD, HARROW, HA1 3UJ

Antibiotic treated hamsters are susceptible to C.difficile infection and disease. We investigated the possibility that prior colonization of hamsters by non-pathogenic strains would protect them from subsequent challenge with a pathogenic strain. This was shown to be the case in an experiment with a small number of animals (1, 2). This work has now been extended and modified to look at the specificity of this protection. All 17 hamsters, that were not protected in this way, died within 48 hours of challenge with the pathogenic strain. Of the 17 'protected' hamsters, one died by day 10 and, of the remainder, 12 survived for 25 days or more. At this point 5 of the animals were sacrificed for analysis of their caecal contents. Five of the remaining 7 survived for more than 30 days and 3 for more than 50 days, at which point the experiment was terminated. If the established non-pathogenic strains were removed by treatment with vancomycin, prior to challenge with the pathogenic strain, no protection was seen. Challenge with heat-killed suspensions of the non-pathogenic strain failed to induce protection, as did attempts to replace the protective strain with other species of clostridia. The non-pathogenic strain would not protect against subsequent challenge with pathogenic clostridia other than C.difficile (i.e. C.spiroforme). These results imply that the protection afforded by the non-pathogenic strain is specific for C.difficile, that it requires the continued presence of the protective strain and that the mechanism operative is probably one of physical exclusion due to occupation of ecological niches, such as mucosal receptor sites, required for the establishment of the pathogenic strain.

240

REFERENCES

1. Borriello SP, Larson HE, Honour P and Barclay FE. 1982.
    Antibiotic-associated diarrhoea and colitis. In Clinical
    Research Centre Report for 1982. Medical Research Council,
    London. p.96-98.

2. Borriello SP. 1983. Clostridium difficile and gut disease. In
    Microbes and Infections of the Gut. Ed. C.S. Goodwin.
    Blackwell Scientific, London. In press.

COLONIZATION RESISTANCE OF THE GASTROINTESTINAL TRACT - A POTENTIAL IN VITRO METHOD FOR THE DETERMINATION OF SUSCEPTIBILITY TO INFECTION WITH CLOSTRIDIUM DIFFICILE

S.P. BORRIELLO, FIONA BARCLAY, A.R. WELCH.   CLINICAL RESEARCH CENTRE, WATFORD ROAD, HARROW, HA1 3UJ.

The normal gut flora is important in protection against gut infections. The administration of antimicrobials results in disruption of the normal gut flora and can predispose to C.difficile infection. An in vitro test system, based on growth in faecal emulsions, has been developed in order to show the importance of the normal gut flora in preventing the establishment of C.difficile in vivo. Cytotoxigenic C.difficile were added to dilutions of stool specimens from 18 healthy adults and 30 patients with antibiotic-associated diarrhoea (AAD) who were negative for C.difficile and its cytotoxin. These were incubated anaerobically for 72 hours and both total and spore counts performed at 24 hour intervals. Toxin and pH levels were also estimated. In parallel, emulsions prepared from normal stools were sterilized by autoclaving or centrifugation and filtration. The results of growth in faecal emulsions, from different patient groups, are shown in the table. Growth of C.difficile was inhibited when in the presence of the faecal flora of healthy volunteers. Sterile faecal emulsions or filtrates of these stool samples were no longer inhibitory, showing the importance of viable bacteria. Eight of the AAD stools failed to inhibit C.difficile. One of these patients subsequently became colonized. The filtrates of 13 of the 22 inhibitory AAD stools were shown to be inhibitory which, probably, reflects inhibitory faecal levels of the offending antibiotic. Stools found to be positive for C.difficile, on original culture, were also tested for their ability to inhibit the organism. In these cases the levels of indigenous C.difficile were measured. No growth inhibition could be demonstrated.

These observations highlight the importance of a normal gut flora in the prevention of disease and indicate that it may be possible to identify those patients at risk by use of an *in vitro* test system. Research is in progress to identify the minimal components of the normal bacterial flora which will confer protection against C.difficile infection, as this offers a more natural alternative to drug therapy.

TABLE

Change in Growth of C.difficile after 48 hours incubation in faecal emulsions

Source of stool sample (No.)	Inhibition of C.difficile	Change in $\log_{10}$ No. C.difficile/ml of faecal emulsion (Range)
Normal (18)	+	-2.6 (-4.2- 0)
Normal, heat sterilized (5)	-	+0.9 (-1.1- 3.8)
Normal, filter sterilized (5)	-	+0.8 (0- 1.5)
C.difficile positive AAD (14)	-	+0.9 (-0.40- 6.0)
C.difficile negative AAD (8)	-	+0.1 (-0.3- 4.0)
C.difficile negative AAD		
(a) Inhibitory filtrate (13)	+	-4.3 (-7.3- -2.8)
(b) Non-inhibitory filtrate (9)	+	-1.2 (-1.7- -0.5)

+ = Inhibition

- = No inhibition

ANAEROBIOSPIRILLUM SPP. FROM ANIMALS AND MAN

H. MALNICK, M.E.M. THOMAS, H. LOTAY, M. ROBBINS. NATIONAL
COLLECTION OF TYPE CULTURES, CENTRAL PUBLIC HEALTH LABORATORY,
COLINDALE AVENUE, LONDON NW9 5HT.

Anaerobiospirilla are anaerobic spiral organisms with bipolar
tufts of flagella. A.succiniproducens was described by Davis et al.
(1) who isolated three similar organisms from beagle dogs. Since
then there have been reports of this organism being recovered from
blood cultures of three febrile adult human patients (2, 3). Of the
three Anaerobiospirillum strains we have tested, two were isolated
during routine diagnostic examination of faeces from patients with
diarrhoea (4) and the third was a strain from puppy faeces.

The prevalence of these organisms in human sites is not
documented, nor is their potential pathogenicity known.
Anaerobiospirillum can be found occasionally in dog and pig faeces
(M.J. Hudson, personal communication) but they have not been studied
closely.

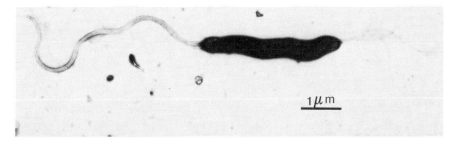

Electron micrograph of Anaerobiospirillum (canine, cultured for
24 hours)

244

REFERENCES

1. Davis CP, Cleven D, Brown J, Balish E. 1976.
    Anaerobiospirillum, a new genus of spiral-shaped bacteria.
    Int.J.Syst.Bacteriol. 26: 498-504.

2. Malnick H, Thomas MEM, Lotay H, Robbins M. 1983.
    Anaerobiospirillum species isolated from humans with diarrhoea.
    J.Clin.Pathol. 36: 1097-1101.

3. Rifkin GD, Opdyke JE, 1981. Anaerobiospirillum succiniproducens
    septicemia. J.Clin.Microbiol. 13: 811-13.

4. Shlaes DM, Dul MJ, Lerner PI. 1982. Anaerobiospirillum
    bacteremia. Ann.Intern.Med. 97: 63-5.

MOTILE CURVED BACILLI ISOLATED FROM THE GENITAL TRACT

M.S. SPROTT, H.R. INGHAM, R.S. PATTMAN*, R.L. EISENSTADT, G.R. SHORT, H.K. NARANG, P.R. SISSON, L.M. CLARKSON AND J.B. SELKON. REGIONAL PUBLIC HEALTH LABORATORY AND *DEPARTMENT OF SEXUALLY TRANSMITTED DISEASES, GENERAL HOSPITAL, NEWCASTLE-UPON-TYNE NE4 6BE

Motile curved bacilli seen in wet preparations of vaginal secretions have been isolated on Columbia agar supplemented with 5% human blood and vitamin K. Growth occurred anaerobically and in 5% oxygen, but not in more aerobic conditions. Morphologically, two types were distinguishable; short curved rods (SCR) 1 - 2 μm in length giving a positive reaction in Gram's stain, and long curved rods (LCR) 2 - 4 μm in length, Gram-variable, but predominantly negative. Electron microscopy revealed that the SCR had 2 - 6 subpolar flagella, with a common point of origin on the concave side. The LCR had flagella arising from several different points.

All strains of the curved rods gave negative results in tests for catalase, oxidase, urease and indole production. Other biochemical reactions are shown in the table.

TABLE

Characteristics of motile curved rods
(Reproduced by kind permission of J.Med.Microbiol.)

Character	Short curved rods	Long curved rods
Growth on 5% human-blood agar	No haemolysis colonies white	α -haemolysis colonies brown
Reaction in Gram's stain	Positive	Variable
ONPG	+	-
Hippurate hydrolysis	+	-
Arginine hydrolysis	+	-
Maltose (Rapid Carbohydrate Utilization Test)	+	-
Reduction of nitrate	+/-	-

All strains were very sensitive to a wide range of antimicrobials, with the exception of nalidixic acid, polymyxin and metronidazole. There was a notable difference between the two groups in their sensitivity to metronidazole, the range of minimum inhibitory concentrations being 0.5 - 4 mg/L for the LCR, but 16 - 1000 mg/L for the SCR.

Motile curved rods were isolated from 18 of 80 patients with a clinical diagnosis of non-specific vaginitis, but from only two of 89 without the disease.

THE PATHOGENESIS OF BACTEROIDES FRAGILIS BACTERAEMIA AND TISSUE LOCALIZATION IN THE MOUSE

S.C. BALDOCK, K.G. McCULLAGH, S. OSWALD AND A.M.S. POPE.
G.D. SEARLE & CO. LTD., P.O.BOX 53, LANE END ROAD, HIGH WYCOMBE,
BUCKS., HP12 4HL.

A non-fatal, biphasic infection developed following i.v. or i.p. inoculation of B.fragilis in mice. A transient bacteraemic phase was followed by localization in various tissues, especially the liver. The degree of the bacteraemia was proportional to the size of the inoculum. Clearance of organisms from the blood, following i.v. infection, was faster than that after i.p. inoculation. No viable B.fragilis were found in blood samples 12 hours after i.v. infection, but were detectable 24 hours after i.p. inoculation. The addition of freeze-dried faeces to i.p. inocula did not affect the level of bacteraemia, but prolonged the period over which B.fragilis could be recovered (up to 48 hours).

Culture of liver homogenates showed that B.fragilis was present for up to 3 days after i.v. infection (maximum 2.6 ± 0.1 $\log_{10}$ cfu/ml at 24 hours). Following i.p. inoculation, organisms were recoverable up to 6 days (maximum 2.3 ± 0.2 $\log_{10}$ cfu/ml at 24 hours). Addition of freeze-dried faeces increased both the number of organisms recovered (5.5 ± 0.13 $\log_{10}$ cfu/ml at 3 days) and the period over which they were detectable (10d).

It was concluded that the sustained bacteraemia occurring after i.p. inoculation results from the continued entry of bacteria from the peritoneal reservoir. The addition of faeces does not affect either the entry rate, or the level of bacteraemia, but prolongs the entry phase, presumably by enhancing the viability of the bacteria. Tissue localization is related to the duration of the bacteraemia rather than to its height.

A COMPARISON BETWEEN THE BACTERIAL FLORA AND OLIGOSACCHARIDE CONTENT OF ILEOSTOMY EFFLUENT IN SUBJECTS TAKING DIETS RICH IN REFINED OR UNREFINED CARBOHYDRATE

S. HORI, LOUISE BERGHOUSE, M. HILL, M. HUDSON, J. LENNARD-JONES AND ELIZABETH ROGERS. PHLS-CAMR, PORTON DOWN, SALISBURY, WILTS AND ST.MARK'S HOSPITAL, CITY ROAD, LONDON EC1

Dietary surveys have shown that more sucrose was eaten by patients with Crohn's disease than by control subjects. The following experiment was undertaken to determine whether a diet rich in refined carbohydrate affects the bacterial flora of the terminal ileum. Ileostomy effluent from 5 patients with Crohn's disease and 5 with ulcerative colitis, after 2 weeks on a diet rich in sucrose (Diet A), has been compared with the same period on a diet rich in unrefined carbohydrate (Diet B). The ten volunteer patients were clinically free of recurrence of disease and were given appropriate dietary advice and their compliance assessed by a trained dietician. Observations were made hourly for 9 hours, after eating equicaloric breakfasts representing the two diets.

The total amount of ileostomy effluent was greater on Diet B than on Diet A both in terms of wet weight (238 ± 89 g vs 162 ± 79 g $p < 0.02$) and dry weight (23.6 ± 6.8 g vs 14.9 ± 6.6 g $p < 0.01$). Surprisingly, the amount of glucose and oligosaccharide in the ileostomy effluent was also greater on Diet B than on Diet A (169 ± 41 mg vs 82 ± 26 mg $p < 0.001$) in all ten volunters.

The bacterial flora (expressed as $\log_{10}$ cfu/gm wet weight of stoma effluent obtained by intubation) was higher on Diet B than on Diet A, at all times following the test breakfast, significantly so after 3 hrs. ($p \quad 0.02$). The table shows selected results for two periods on the two diets.

	3-4 hours		5-6 hours	
	Diet A	Diet B	Diet A	Diet B
Total Flora	6.5±1.1	7.2±1.1**	6.8±1.2	7.5±1.4**
Facultative Anaerobes	6.5±1.2	7.2±1.0**	6.8±1.1	7.3±1.4
Streptococci	6.3±1.1	7.0±1.0**	6.5±1.0	7.3±1.5**
Enterococci	5.4±1.3	6.2±1.1**	6.1±1.2	6.8±1.5**
Enterobacteria	3.9±1.5	4.8±2.1	4.7±1.6	5.4±1.9
Lactobacilli	3.5±1.9	4.3±1.6	3.6±1.2	4.6±1.4
Obligate Anaerobes	5.0±1.2	5.4±1.5	5.0±1.6	5.4±2.1
Bacteroides spp.	3.2±1.2	3.5±1.7	3.2±1.1	3.8±1.8
Veillonellae	4.5±1.2	4.8±1.6	4.2±1.4	5.1±2.0
Clostridium spp.	3.9±1.6	3.9±1.5	3.9±1.5	4.4±1.9

(** $p < 0.05$ by Paired 't' test Diet A < Diet B)

Diet B appeared to favour a greater flora, due to a general increase in all of the organisms and not through qualitative changes of species. Obligate anaerobes, predominantly bacteroides, veillonellae and clostridia, were also more common in the fasting ileum of patients consuming Diet B. No differences were detected between patients with ulcerative colitis and those with Crohn's disease and the above study does not support the hypothesis that the latter disease is due to an overgrowth of specific bacteria in the terminal ileum.

INFLUENCE OF DIETARY LACTOSE AND AGE ON THE METABOLIC ACTIVITY OF
THE RAT CAECAL MICROFLORA

A.K. MALLETT AND I.R. ROWLAND AND A. WISE.   BIBRA AND MRC TOXICOLOGY
LABORATORIES, CARSHALTON, SURREY SM5 4DS

Weanling (3 wk old) or adult (9 wk old) LAC : P rats were
randomised into three groups for each age and fed a purified,
fibre-free diet, or the same diet incorporating lactose (250 or
500 g/kg diet) at the expense of glucose. After 10 days treatment,
various caecal parameters and microbial enzyme activities
(azoreductase, β-glucosidase, β-glucuronidase, nitrate reductase,
nitroreductase and urease) were determined.

Adult rats, fed the control diet, had larger caeca than
weanlings, but the total number of bacteria was not significantly
different. Total caecal nitrate reductase activity was greatest in
control weanling animals, while urease activity was greatest in
control adults. When enzyme activities were expressed per kg
bodyweight, values were generally lower in adults.

Lactose treatment increased the weight of caecal contents and
increased significantly the total caecal bacterial population in
both age groups, yet decreased the concentration of organisms
(per g) in weanlings. Lactose increased significantly nitrate
reductase activity in both age groups, and decreased azoreductase
and nitroreductase activity in weanlings. Urease activity also
increased in both age groups in response to lactose, with a
concomitant increase in total ammonia content. Animals fed lactose
had caecal contents of lower pH (5.9-6.7) than control animals
(7.8-8.1) for both age groups.

This study demonstrates that caecal microbial enzyme activities differ in weanling and adult rats given a control diet. These differences may be of toxicological importance in the young animals due to the higher anzyme activity in relation to bodyweight. The differential response of young and old animals to lactose, suggests an age-dependent variation in the strain or species composition of the gut ecosystem.

This work was supported in part by the U.K. Ministry of Agriculture, Fisheries and Food, to whom AKM and IRR express their thanks. The results are Crown Copywright.

THE EFFECT OF DIET ON THE COMPOSITION OF THE BACTERIAL FLORA ON THE
TERMINAL ILEUM

F. FERNANDEZ, H. KENNEDY, M. HILL AND S. TRUELOVE. BACTERIAL
METABOLISM RESEARCH LABORATORY, PHLS CENTRE FOR APPLIED MICROBIOL.
AND RESEARCH, PORTON DOWN, SALISBURY, WILTS. SP4 OJG and RADCLIFFE
INFIRMARY, OXFORD

It is known from _in vitro_ studies that the nutrient source is
important in determining the composition of mixed bacterial
populations and so it has been assumed that the total colonic
bacterial flora is related to diet. Studies of the faecal flora
have not shown such a relation, but it has been suggested that the
flora of the right colon may be more sensitive to changes in
nutrients (1). We have studied the bacterial flora of the ileostomy
effluent of 11 patients who had all undergone total colectomy for
ulcerative colitis many years ago. Samples were collected fresh
from the stoma and stored in cryoprotective broth until
bacteriological analysis was performed by the methods of Borriello
_et al_ (2). The patients were sampled on a control diet and after
two week periods on a low protein ($40-50g.d^{-1}$) high protein (more
than $120g.d^{-1}$), low fat ($40-50g.d^{-1}$) and high fat (more than
$120g.d^{-1}$) diet.

The ileostomy flora was similar during the control period, the
low fat (LF) and the low protein (LP) diets (Table) and there were
no statistically different counts of any organisms except
Veillonella spp (which almost disappeared during the low protein
diet) and bifidobacteria (which disappeared during the low fat
diet). A high protein (HP) diet resulted in increased numbers of
the total aerobes ($P < 0.01$), enterobacteria ($P. < 0.05$), streptococci
($P < 0.05$), and lactobacilli ($P < 0.001$) in comparison with either
control or low protein diets and of _Veillonella_ spp in comparison
with the low protein diet ($P < 0.05$). A high fat (HF) diet caused an
increase in total anaerobes ($P < 0.05$), lactobacilli ($P < 0.05$) and
Bacteroides spp.

TABLE   Viable organisms ($\log_{10}$gm^{-1} wet weight)

Organism	C Diet	LP Diet	HP Diet	LF Diet	HF Diet
Tot. Aerobes	5.7	5.7	6.7	5.7	6.2
Tot. Anaerobes	4.5	4.7	4.9	4.9	5.6
Enterobact.	4.5	4.3	6.0	4.2	5.3
Streptococci	5.6	5.1	6.3	5.5	5.6
Enterococci	2.9(7/11)	2.7(6/11)	4.2(7/10)	3.6(8/9)	3.9(8/9)
Lactobacilli	0 (0/11)	0.3(1/11)	3.7(8/10)	0.5(1/9)	1.9(4/9)
Bacteroides	3.7(9/11)	3.0(7/11)	4.1(8/10)	3.5(8/9)	4.8(8/9)
Bifidobact.	1.4	0.9	1.8	0	1.8
Clostridia	3.8	3.3	3.6	4.2	4.7
Veillonella	2.0(7/11)	0.5(2/11)	2.6(5/10)	2.0(4/9)	1.9(4/9)

The total number of organisms per g. ileostomy effluent was 10^5 during the control, LF and LP diets and 10^6 during the HP and HF diets. Bacteroides spp were isolated from 7/11 during the LP diet, 8/10 on HP and 8/9 on LF and HF. In contrast, lactobacilli were not detected in any patient during the control period and in only 1/11 on LP and 1/9 on LF compared with 8/10 on HP and 4/9 on HF diet.

Clearly the bacterial flora of ileostomy fluid does not represent that of the normal caecum, but it must be closer than that of faeces. These results suggest that the diet has a profound effect on the bacterial flora of the distal ileum and probably also on the proximal colon.

REFERENCES

1. Hill MJ. (1981) in "Colon and Nutrition" (ed H. Kaspar and H. Goebell) HTP, Lancaster p37-45.
2. Borriello SP, Hudson MJ and Hill MJ. 1978; in Clinics in Gastroenterology 7, 329-49. London, W.B. Saunders.

STEROID DEGRADATION IN THE GASTROINTESTINAL TRACT - THE USE OF
CANNULATED PIGS AS A MODEL SYSTEM

K. FADDEN, R.W. OWEN, M.J. HILL, E. LATYMER, G. LOW, A.N. MASON
BACTERIAL METABOLISM RESEARCH LABORATORY, PHLS CENTRE FOR APPLIED
MICROBIOLOGY AND RESEARCH, PORTON DOWN, SALISBURY, WILTS, S4 OJG.

It has been postulated that the right colon may be the most
important site for the microbial degradation of steroids in man
(1). The extent of bile acid degradation from the terminal ileum to
the rectum is important in that this will determine the
concentration of secondary bile acids (e.g. deoxycholic acid (DCA)
and lithocholic acid (LCA)) present within the lumen. Numerous
studies have shown DCA and LCA to be co-mutagenic and/or
co-carcinogenic (2). The cannulated pig was used as a model system
to obtain a profile of acid and neutral steroids along the
gastro-intestinal tract. However the major primary bile acids in
the pig are hyocholic acid (HCA), and chenodeoxycholic acid (CDCA)
which are dehydroxylated to hyodeoxycholic acid (HDCA) and LCA
respectively.

Three Landrace x Large white boars were fitted with simple gut
cannulas in the ileum, caecum and mid colon. Digesta samples plus
faeces were collected and extracted using the Sochlet method (3).
Each extract was subsequently fractionated using DEAP-LH-20 column
chromatography (3), and quantitated by gas-liquid-chromatography.

Results of the study (Table 1) indicated that extensive
metabolism of steroids occurs within the caecum; values for
deconjugation and 7α-dehydroxylation of bile acids and reduction of
cholesterol within the caecum are in the range 59-99%. Further
metabolism throughout the large intestine is between 1% and 14%.

There is, however considerable bile acid deconjugation in the ileum (56%), this is probably a result of the pig anterior gut being colonized, by Coliform, Lactobacillus and Streptococcus species at mean $\log_{10}$ viable counts of between 6.8 and 8.8 (4). Faecal values for percentage conversions of CDCA and cholesterol are comparable to human studies. Thus, in certain respects, steroid metabolism in the pig has many similarities to man.

Table 1. Percentage conversions of steroids along the gastrointestinal tract

Substrate	Enzyme	Product	Percentage Conversion			
			Ileum	Caecum	Colon	Faeces
Cholesterol	Cholesterol Reductase	Coprostanol	1	59	56	67
CDCA	7 Dehydrox-ylase	LCA	6	84	93	98
Conjugated Bile Acid	Bile Acid Conjugate Hydrolase	Free Bile Acids (HDCA + CDCA)	56	99	100	100

In conclusion, the cannulated pig may be considered a reasonable model system, which implicates the caecum and, therefore, the right colon as the most important site for microbial degradation of steroids.

REFERENCES

1. Hill MJ. (1982), Colonic Bacterial Activity in: Dietary Fibre in Health and Disease. GV Vahouny and D. Kritchevsky, Eds., New York Plenum Press, pp 35-43.
2. Reddy BS, Watanabe K, (1979), Effect of cholesterol metabolites and Promoting effect of Lithocholic Acid in Colon Carcinogenesis in Germ-Free and Conventional F344 Rats. Cancer Research, 39, 1521-1524.

256

3. Owen RW, et al., (1981), Analysis of Metabolic Profiles of Bile Acids in Faeces of Patients Undergoing Chenodeoxycholic Acid Therapy Using Liquid-Gel Chromatographic Techniques and Gas-Liquid Chromatography - Mass Spectrometry. Falk Symposium 31, Colonic Carcinogenesis.

4. Barrow PA, Fuller R, Newport MJ. (1977), Changes in the Microflora and Physiology of the Anterior Intestinal Tract of Pigs Weaned at 2 days, with Special Reference to the Pathogenesis of Diarrhea. Infection and Immunity 18, 586-595.

THE ESTABLISHMENT OF COMPLEX COMMUNITIES OF ORAL BACTERIA IN THE CHEMOSTAT USING MULTIPLE, DEFINED INOCULA

ANN S. McDERMID, AILSA S. McKEE, P.D. MARSH AND D.C. ELLWOOD.
PATHOGENIC MICROBES RESEARCH LABORATORY, PHLS CENTRE FOR APPLIED
MICROBIOLOGY AND RESEARCH, PORTON DOWN, SALISBURY, WILTS SP4 OJG.

Dental plaque is a complex microbial community containing a high species diversity. In plaque, gradients of ecologically significant factors develop and influence the bacterial growth. This will result in the bacteria growing at sub-maximal rates, due to a range of nutrient limitations. Recently, it has been shown that, in line with chemostat theory, complex, mixed, interacting cultures could be established in a chemostat inoculated with dental plaque (1). Consequently, we have investigated the possibility of establishing reproducible communities in chemostats using defined inocula. In this way we hope to obtain further information about the biochemical properties of oral bacterial populations, and the nature of some of the interactions between different species. Strains of Lactobacillus casei, Streptococcus sanguis, S.mutans, S.mitior, Veillonella alkalescens, Neisseria sp. Fusobacterium nucleatum, Bacteroides intermedius and Actinomyces viscosus, were inoculated into a chemostat before it was put on flow in a complex medium at pH 7.0 and a dilution rate of 0.05 h^{-1} (MGT = 14 h) under a gas phase of 95% nitrogen and 5% carbon dioxide. In a glucose-limited chemostat, all the above species established whereas S.mutans, B.intermedius and Neisseria sp., were unable to persist under amino-acid limitation (glucose-excess). Three inoculations were necessary to establish some of the bacterial species. Preliminary studies suggest that duplicate chemostat experiments, using identically prepared inocula, result in the establishment of communities of similar composition and are not simply a reproduction of the inocula. The table illustrates the steady-state populations found in the chemostats under glucose-limited and glucose-excess conditions.

The standard deviations are calculated from daily counts performed over a period of approximately one month. In most cases, these are low, whereas those for S.mutans and A.viscosus are higher due to difficulties in their detection and identification. Run A and run B represent independent duplicate chemostats.

TABLE

BACTERIAL SPECIES	LOG COUNT VALUE + S.D.			
	GLUCOSE-LIMITED CHEMOSTAT		GLUCOSE-EXCESS CHEMOSTAT	
	RUN A	RUN B	RUN A	RUN B
L.casei	7.7+0.19	8.2+0.56	9.1+0.05	8.9+0.34
S.sanguis	7.0+1.38	7.2+0.87	7.4+0.45	6.7+1.12
S.mutans	6.4+0.60	5.0+4.95	N.D.	N.D.
S.mitior	9.1+0.16	8.4+0.70	7.1+0.25	7.2+0.63
V.alkalescens	8.2+0.48	8.5+0.47	8.5+0.02	9.1+0.56
Neisseria sp.	2.9+1.50	3.7+0.79	N.D.	N.D.
B.intermedius	6.8+0.54	7.5+0.52	N.D.	N.D.
F.nucleatum	7.5+0.51	7.5+0.24	6.8+0.52	6.8+0.56
A.viscosus	7.5+0.51	5.3+2.14	7.2+3.20	7.8+0.50

N.D. represents not detected.

The proportions of species in the bacterial community adhering to the walls of the culture vessel differed from that in the liquid medium, and also varied between sites with different environmental conditions, i.e. if the site was above or below, or at, the liquid-gas interface. Microscopic examination of the communities in the chemostat and of single colonies on primary isolation plates provided evidence for some specific species interactions. Acid production by oral communities is a major virulence factor in dental caries, (which is one of the most prevalent diseases affecting western man). Fermentation products and acid production by washed cells differed with the growth limitation. Generally, more acid was produced by washed cells from the glucose-excess chemostat, which is in contrast to studies using mono-cultures. The results obtained in this study are in general agreement with those obtained when dental plaque was the inoculum. This indicates that the chemostat could make a valuable contribution to the study of the ecology of oral bacteria.

REFERENCE

1. Marsh et al. 1983. J.Gen.Microbiol. 129: 755.

ENHANCEMENT OF EXPERIMENTAL ULCERATIVE COLITIS BY IMMUNIZATION WITH BACTEROIDES VULGATUS

R. CISNEROS AND A.B. ONDERDONK. TUFTS UNIVERSITY SCHOOL OF VETERINARY MEDICINE, 305 SOUTH STREET, JAMAICA PLAIN, MASS.02130, USA

Studies using the guinea pig model for ulcerative colitis have shown that the inducing agent, carrageenan (C), did not induce ulcerations when fed to germfree guinea pigs. Mono-association of germfree guinea pigs with Bacteroides vulgatus, prior to feeding C, resulted in the development of caecal ulcerations in all animals. Immunization of guinea pigs with B.vulgatus resulted in circulating antibody levels and positive skin tests. Immune animals were given either C alone, fed B.vulgatus daily, or administered C and live B.vulgatus concurrently. Immunized animals fed C or C and B.vulgatus developed ulcerations of the caecum and entire large intestine within 21 days, but lesions were more severe in the latter group. Animals fed B.vulgatus alone did not develop ulcerations, but showed histological evidence of inflammation. Control animals receiving C did not develop lesions as severe as comparable immune groups. Lesions observed in immune animals were most severe in the colon and rectum, in contrast to more severe caecal lesions seen in non-immune controls. Similar experiments with B.fragilis showed no difference between immune and non-immune groups. These results indicate that immunization with B.vulgatus enhances the severity of induced ulcerative colitis.

INTRODUCTION TO THE SOCIETY FOR INTESTINAL MICROBIAL ECOLOGY
AND DISEASE

A series of symposia concerned with intestinal microbial ecology
and its relation to various intestinal and other diseases has been
held in the United States every other year for some 15 years. The
first six were held at the University of Missouri Medical School,
columbia, Mo. and the VII and VIII International Microecology
Symposia were held in 1982 and 1983 in Boston with Tufts University
School of Medicine and School of Veterinary Medicine serving as host
(together with the University of Missouri, Columbia in 1982 and
SIMED in 1983).

At the 1982 Executive Committee meeting of the Intestinal
Microecology Group (an informally constituted group that ran these
meetings), there was unanimous agreement that we should set up a
formal society as soon as possible. Dr. Don Luckey appointed Dr.
Dave Hentges, Dr. Dwayne Savage and me as an Organizing Committee.

At the 1983 meeting, our society was formally constituted. We
chose the name Society for Intestinal Microbial Ecology and Disease
and the abbreviated name SIMED. Officers elected at the 1983
meeting were S.M. Finegold, President, D.C. Savage, Secretary and
D.J. Hentges, Treasurer. A nominating committee headed by Victor
Bokkenheuser will recommend candidates for the President-Elect and
Councillors and these will be voted on. The aims of the society are
to foster training, research and disseminiation of knowledge
concerning intestinal microbial ecology and its relation to
disease. Membership is open to anyone anywhere in the world who has
an interest in one or more of the aims of the society. There are
three categories of membership -- regular (annual dues $25),
student, including pre-doctoral and post-doctoral fellows (annual
dues $10) and corporate (minimum annual dues $250). There is no
initiation fee. Eventually we expect to be set up as a tax exempt
non-profit corporation. A Constitution and By-Laws have been
developed.

Sydney M. Finegold, M.D.

ABSTRACTS OF THE FIRST MEETING
OF THE SOCIETY FOR INTESTINAL MICROBIAL ECOLOGY
AND DISEASE, BOSTON, MASSACHUSETTS, 1983

LIST OF ABSTRACTS

V. Bokkenheuser, MD.,
St.Luke's Roosevelt Hospital Centre,
Amsterdam Avenue at 114th Street, New York, NY 10025

Title of Abstract: (1)   "Microflora-A Potential Marker Colerectal
                          Cancer"

Michael Stek, Jr. MD.,
Uniformed Services University of the Health Sciences, School of
Medicine, 4301 Jones Bridge Road, Bethesda, MD 20814

Title of Abstract: (2)   "Malabsorption, Enterocyte, Kinetics, Tropical
                          Sprue, and Giardiasis"

Charles E. Edminston, Jr.Ph.D.,
University of Wisconsin-Parkside, Box 2000, Kenosha, WI 53141

Title of Abstract: (3)   "Fiberoptic Colonoscopy: An In Vivo Biopsy
                          Technique for Investigating Anaerobic Micro-
                          ecology"

Adrian Soerjadi-Liem, Ph.D.,
University of Massachusetts, Department of Veterinary and Animal
Sciences, Paige Laboratory, Amherst, MA 01003

Title of Abstract: (4)   "Bacterial interference and possible mode of
                          action by native gut microflora in limiting
                          infections by some enteric pathogens in
                          chickens"

C.D. Nord, R. Bennet, M. Eriksson and R. Zetterstrom,
Department of Pediatrics, St. Goran's Children's Hospital, Department
of Microbiology, Huddinge University Hospital, Karolinska Institute,
and National Bacteriological Laboratory, Stockholm, Sweden.

Title of Abstract: (5)   "Impact of Gentamicin and Ampicillin Treatment
                          on the Colon Microflora in Newborns"

Yoshimi Benno, DVM, PhD.,
Riken, Institute of Physical and Chemical Research, Wako, Saitama, 351,
Japan.

Title of Abstract: (6)   "The Fecal Bacterial Flora of Infants with
                          Vitamin K Deficiency"

Kunihiko Suzuki, MD.,
Third Department of Internal Medicine, Tokoku University School of
Medicine, 1-1 Seiryo-machi, Sendai, Japan 980.

Title of Abstract: (7)   "Fecal Flora of Patients with Crohn's Disease
                          Untreated and treated with Elemental Diet"

Gerald L. Larsen,
P.O. Box 5674, State University Station, Fargo, ND 58105.

Title of Abstract: (8) "Catabolism and Potential Retoxication of
Mercapturic Acid Pathway Metabolites of
Xenobiotics in the Gastrointestinal Tract"

M.J. Allison, H.M. Cook, C.A. Thorne and R.V. Clayman
National Animal Disease Center, ARS, USDA, Ames, IA 50010

Title of Abstract: (9) "Loss of Oxalate-Degrading Bacteria From the
Colon: An Hypothesis to Explain Enteric
Hyperoxaluria"

Charalabos Pathoulakis, MD.
University Hospital, 75 EastNewton Street, Boston, MA 02118.

Title of Abstract: (10) "Effects of Clostridium Difficile Toxin B on
Macromolecular Synthesis in Human Lung
Fibroblasts and Cecal Epithelial Cells"

Meyer J. Wolin, Ph.D.
State of New York Department of Health, Tower Building, Governor Nelson
A. Rockefeller Empire State Plaza, Albany, NY 12201.

Title of Abstract: (11) "Methanogens and total anaerobes in a colon
segment isolated from the normal fecal stream"

J. Robert Cantey, MD.,
Veterans Administration Medical Center, 109, Bee Street, Charleston SC
29403.

Title of Abstract: (12) "Pili mediate the ability of Escherichia coli
(RDEC-1) bacteria to adhere, but not persist,
on rabbit ileal lymph follicle epithelium"

Kenneth H. Wilson MD.
Division of Infectious Diseases, Veterans Administration Medical
Center, 2215 Fuller Road, Ann Arbor, MI 48105.

Title of Abstract:(13) "Association of Germfree Mice with Conventional
Hamster Flora"

H.M. Cowley
Department of Microbiology, University of Witwatersand, 1, Jan Smuts
Avenue, Braafontein, Johannesburg, 2001, South Africa.

Title of Abstract: (14) "Spirochetes of the Rat Gastroentestinal Tract"

S.P. Borriello,
Clinical Research Centre, Watford Road, Harrow, Middlesex, HA1 3UJ.

Title of Abstract: (15) "Lignan Production by Faecal Flora"
(16) "Colonization resistance of the
gastrointestinal tract - a potential in vitro
method for the determination of susceptibility
to infection with C.difficile"

K. Ramotar, J. Conly, E. Bow, A. Ronald and T.J. Louie
University of Manitoba, Winnipeg, Canada.

Title of Abstract: (17) "Correlation of Hypoprothrobinemia with Suppression of Menaquinone Producing Intestinal Microflora"

R.J. Carman, S.P. Borriello and A.B. Price.
Charing Cross Hospital Medical School, St. Dunstan's Road, London W6 8RP, England.

Title of Abstract: (18) "Rabbit Enterotoxaemia: Characteristics of Clostridium Spiroforme and its Toxin.

MICROFLORA - A POTENTIAL MARKER FOR COLORECTAL CANCER

Jeanette Winter and Victor D. Bokkenheuser - St. Luke's - Roosevelt Hospital Center, New York, NY 10025.

During enterohepatic circulation conjugated steroids are hydrolyzed by intestinal bacteria, further metabolized mainly by anaerobic bacteria, reabsorbed, reconjugated and delivered to the blood for renal excretion. 21-Dehydroxlylation of tetrahydrodeoxycorticosterone (THCOD) to pregnanolone is performed exclusively by Eubacterium lentum, a normal inhabitant of the intestinal flora. The concentration of E. lentum in feces can be determined from the highest dilution of fresh voided stool capable of 21-dehydroxylating THDOC. Such studies revealed that the concentration increases from 10^6/g wet feces during the first year of life to 10^8/g feces in the 7th and 8th decade. Colonization appears to be independent of diet since the organisms are present in babies whether breast-fed or on formula, in subjects on a "Western diet" and in Africans consuming a diet low in meat and fat.

The steroid metabolite, pregnanolone, biosynthesized by E. lentum is non-carcinogenic in the hamster embryo cell transformation (HECT) test is contrast to its precursor, THDOC. Thus, E. lentum converts a carcinogen to a non-carcinogen.

The concentration of E. lentum in patients with sigmoidal and rectal cancer (60-80 years of age) was 10^5/g wet feces which is less than 1% of the mean for the same age group of "normals" (p 0.05). Patients with colonic polyps showed also significantly lower concentrations of 21-dehydroxylating bacteria than did "normals" but higher than the patients with distal colorectal cancern.

The data suggest that the concentration of 21-dehydroxylating bacteria in freshly voided feces is a potential marker for colorectal cancer.

MALABSORPTION, ENTEROCYTE KINETICS, TROPICAL SPRUE, AND GIARDIASIS

Michael Stek, Jr., Division of Tropical Public Health, Department of
Preventive Medicine and Biometrics, Uniformed Services University of
the Health Sciences, Bethesda, Maryland 20814.

Giardiasis may leas to fat malabsorption and protein loss as
well as decreases in vitamins A, D, E, K, B_{12}, and folate, and the
enzymes xylase and lactase. Stool fat, D-xylose and lactose
tolerance tests, and serum A, B_{12}, and folate levels were used as
measures of malabsorption in 16 giardiasis patients. The severity
of disease was found to be increased in those regurning from sojourn
to countries where tropical sprue was prevalent. Jejunal biopsies
were done on 5 giardiasis patients and compared with 3 tropical
sprue patients. Enterocyte kinetics in giardiasis, associated with
progressively severe villus changes, were shown to correspond with
the tropical sprue histologic data. Crypt size, morphology and
number of mitoses were noted to be similar for the 2 groups. An 80%
cure rate of giardiasis with metronidazole was found for the 16
giardiasis patients. The recovery time of 4-10 days for the
restoration of relatively normal intestinal absorptive capacity in
these patients correlated with the expected enterocyte turnover time
of 3-8 days. This work indicated that enterocyte kinetics were
important in the pathophysiology of malabsorption as seen in
giardiasis. Further, although Giardia may occur as a concomitant
infection with tropical sprue, it is also possible that this
intestinal protozoan may be one of the etiologic agents for the
tropical sprue syndrome.

270

FIBEROPTIC COLONOSCOPY: AN <u>IN VIVO</u> BIOPSY TECHNIQUE FOR
INVESTIGATING ANAEROBIC COLONIC MICROECOLOGY.

Charles E. Edmiston, Jr., Allied Health Discipline, University of
Wisconsin-Parkside, Kenosha, WI 53141

Multiple biopsies were obtained from 32 patients during the
course of this study. A total of 114 biopsies representing normal
mucosa were cultured anaerobically. Mucosal epithelium for culture
was obtained from the ascending (ASCD-27), transverse (TRNV-29),
descending (DESCD-38) and sigmoid (SIGM-20) colon. Specimens for
culture were processed and anaerobic isolates were characterized as
previously described (Edmiston et al. J. Infect. Dis. 140:358,
1979). Biopsies were obtained under anaerobic conditions by CO_2
insufflation and sheath biopsy probes as described earlier (Edmiston
et al. Appl. Environ. Microbiol. 43:1173, 1982). Additional
biopsies were used for TEM and SEM evaluation. Mean mucosal weight
values (mg wet weight) + SE for the ASCD, TRNV, DESCD, and SIGM were
4.2 $\pm$ 0.4, 5.1 $\pm$ 0.5, 4.8 $\pm$ 0.3, and 4.4 $\pm$ 0.5, respectively. No
significant difference was observed in biopsy sample size between
the 4 regions. Mean values and (range) for the total number of
organisms from the normal ASCD, TRNV, DESCD, and SIGM were 6.8
(2.5-7.9), 6.3 (2.7-6.9), 7.1 (3.0-7.5) and 5.6 (3.7-6.0) log/mg,
respectively. No difference was seen in mean values between the
ASCD and the other regions studied. Mean values $\pm$ SE for genera
recovered from the ASCD, TRNV, DESCD, and SIGM were 3.2 $\pm$ 0.5, 3.5 $\pm$
0.4, 2.4 $\pm$ 0.3, and 1.9 $\pm$ 0.6, respectively. Mean species recovery
$\pm$ SE from the ASCD, TRNV, DESCD, and SIGM were 5.1 $\pm$ 0.8, 4.9 $\pm$ 0.5,
6.0 $\pm$ 0.5, and 3.5 $\pm$ 0.6, respectively. Genera and species recovery
in the sigmoid was the only region to demonstrate a significant
difference when compared to the ascending colon (p 0.05). The
results of the study suggest that fiberoptic colonoscopy can be
utilized as an innovative probe for studying colonic mucosal flora
<u>in vivo</u>.

BACTERIAL INTERFERENCE AND POSSIBLE MODE OF ACTION BY NATIVE GUT
MICROFLORA IN LIMITING INFECTIONS BY SOME ENTERIC PATHOGENS IN
CHICKENS

A.S. Soerjadi-Liem, G.H. Snoeyenbos and O.M. Weinack Department of
Veterinary and Animal Sciences, University of Massachusets,
Ameherst, Massachusetts 01003.

It has been established that a complex gut microflora, which has
been maintained in a population of specific-pathogen-free chickens,
prevents colonization by paratyphoid salmonellae in young chicks.
Protection is demonstrable 2 hours after dosing chicks with the
microflora and is maximal by 32 hours. Protection is overwhelmed by
massive exposure of salmonellae.

In holoxenic chicks that were infected with Salmonella, major
colonization was demonstrated in the crop and ceca, while in the
absence of other bacterial flora, Salmonella adhered to all regions
of the gastrointestinal tract. Such colonization was stable during
test periods as long as 35 days, with persistent shedding and
bacteremia. Introduction of protective bacteria to either holoxenic
or axenic chicks that had been infected with Salmonella abbreviated
colonization by this pathogen.

In newly-hatched chicks, introduction of this protective
bacteria resulted in early development of a mat of microflora on the
cecal epithelium. Although native gut microflora may protect the
gut by a concert of actions, development of this mat of microflora
is probably the main mechanism of protection.

Subsequent work in this laboratory has shown that colonization
by other enteric pathogens including enteropathogenic Escherichia
coli, campylobacter fetus subsp. jejuni, Clostridium botulinium type
C, Clostridium perfringens type C and Yersinia enterocolitica is
similarly limited by native gut microflora.

IMPACT OF GENTAMICIN AND AMPICILLIN TREATMENT ON THE COLON MICROFLORA IN NEWBORNS

C.E. Nord, R. Bennet, M. Eriksson and R. Zetterstrom, Department of Pediatrics, St. Goran's Children's Hospital, Department of Microbiology, Huddinge University Hospital, Karolinska Institute, and National Bacteriological Laboratory, Stockholm, Sweden.

The immediate effect of parenteral gentamicin and ampicillin in the aerobic and anaerobic colon flora of 14 infants with suspected or proven neonatal septicaemia was studied. Eight infants of similar gestational and postnatal age were studied for comparison. All control infants showed an abundant growth of both aerobic and anaerobic bacteria as early as the first two weeks of life. The treated infants generally had lower counts of aerobic and especially of anaerobic bacteria; in 10 of 16 cultures no anaerobes were isolated. In relation to aerobic strains Escherichia coli dominated in untreated infants and Klebsiella pneumoniae in treated ones.

THE FECAL BACTERIAL FLORA OF INFANTS WITH VITAMIN K DEFICIENCY

Yoshimi Benno[1], Ken Sawade[2] and Tomotari Mitsuoka[1,3], The
Institute of Physical and Chemical Research, Wako, Saitama, 351[1],
Department of Pediatriacs, Toho University School of Medicine,
Ohota-ku, Toxyo, 143[2], and Department of Biomedical Science,
Faculty of Agriculture, University of Tokyo, Bunkyo-ku, Tokyo,
113[3], Japan.

The fecal bacterial flora of ten breast-fed infants with vitamin
K deficiency from 3 to 6-week-old and ten clinically healthy
breast-fed infants of 4-week-old was examined.

Most prominent and meaninfgul findings were the higher frequency
of isolation and counts of Bacteroides species (especially B.
fragilis group) in the infants with vitamin K deficiency. The
counts of Villonella parvula, Escherichia coli and Streptococcus
faecium in the feces of vitamin K deficiency group were increased.
Conversely, the numbers of Bifidobacterium spp. (especially B.
longum) and of Clostridium spp. in their stools were in lower than
those of healthy subjects.

The data suggest that Bacteroides spp. (especially B. fragilis
group) isolated from the fece of infants with vitamin K deficiency
may be closely related to the incidence and promotion of this
disease in the breast-fed infants.

FECAL FLORA OF PATIENTS WITH CROHN'S DISEASE UNTREATED AND TREATED
WITH ELEMENTAL DIET

Kunihiko Suzuki, Hiroshi Hirakawa, Nobuo Hiwatashi, Akio Nagasaki
and Yosio Goto, The Third Department of Internal Medicine, Tohoku
University School of Medicine, Sendai, Japan.

Fecal flora of patients with untreated Crohn's disease were
analysed qualitatively and quantitatively. In comparison with
normal healthy subjects, the counts of bacteroidaceae,
bifidobacteria, clostridia except Clostridium perfringens were
remarkably decreased (p 0.01), while the counts of aerobes
including enterobacteriaceae, micrococcaceae (p 0.01), and
streptococci (p 0.05) were significantly increased. These results
were considered to be secondary changes due to diarrhoea rather than
specific patterns of Crohn's disease.

Changes in fecal flora during treatment with elemental diet
(ED), averaging fifty-five days in patients with Crohn's disease,
were also studied. During treatment with ED the bacterial counts
per gram of wet feces were greater compared with those after
begining of oral digestion. However, average fecal volume per day
during treatment was much smaller than after treatment. It was
concluded that total intestinal bacterial counts were decreased
during treatment. Following treatment with ED, possible harmful
changes of intestinal flora were noted. Especially, clostridia
except Clostridium perfringens were significantly increased.

CATABOLISM AND POTENTIAL RETOXICATION OF MERCAPTURIC ACID PATHWAY
METABOLITES OF XENOBIOTICS IN THE GASTROINTESTINAL TRACT
G.L. Larsen and J.E. Bakke USDA, ARS, Metabolism and Radiation
Research Lab. Fargo, N. D. 58105

To study the metabolism of mercapturic acid pathway (MAP)
metabolites of exnobiotics in the gastrointestinal (GI) tract
MAP-metabolites of propachlor were incubated with GI contents from
the rat and pig and with pure cultures of GI bacteria. Results from
these studies indicate that MAP-metabolites of propachlor were
catabolized to the cysteine conjugate in the GI tract and that a
bacterial enzyme cleaved the cysteine conjugate of propachlor to
2-mercapto-N-isopropylacetanilide. This enzyme has been isolated,
partially purified and characterized as a cysteine conjugate
-lyase from Fusobacterium necrophorum. The enzyme has also been
isolated from other GI bacteria. The cysteine conjugate   -lyase
was shown to cleave the thioether linkage in cysteine conjugates of
S-alkyl (e.g. 2-S-cysteinyl-N-isopropylacetanilide and
1,2-dihydro-1- of S-alkyl (e.g. 2-S-cysteinyl-N-isopropylacetanilide
and 1,2-dihydro-1-hydroxy-2-Scysteinylnapthalene) and S-aryl / e.g.,
S-benzothiazolylcysteine / linked xenobiotics. This enzyme is a
different enzyme than the liver cysteine conjugate   -lyase because
the liver enzyme reportedly only cleaves the thioether linkage in
cysteine conjugates of S-aryl linked xenobiotics. The cleavage of
biliary MAP-metabolites of zenobiotics results in the formation of
thiols in the GI tract. These thiols are precursors for the
formation of nonextractable fecal residues or are excreted as
metabolites of xenobiotics containing methylthio, methylsulfinyl or
methylsulfonyl groups. The toxicology of this pathway is not known.

LOSS OF OXALATE-DEGRADING BACTERIA FROM THE COLON: AN HYPOTHESIS TO
EXPLAIN ENTERIC HYPEROXALURIA

M.J. Allison[1], H.M. Cook[1], C.A. Thorne[2], and R.V. Clayman[2],
National animal Disease Centre, ARS, USDA, Amea, IA 50010[1]; and
V.A. Medical Center, Minneapolis, MN 55417[2]

Hyperoxaluria, with increased risk for urinary stone formation,
is a frequent complication of inflammation or resection of the small
bowel and jejunoileal (JI) bypass surgery for morbid obesity. This
enteric hyperoxaluria is now known to be due to increased colonic
absorption of dietary oxalate.

Proposals to describe a mechanism for enteric hyperoxaluria have
generally centered around altered bile acid metabolism. We propose
that oxalate-degrading bacteria in the colon may significantly
affect concentrations of soluble oxalate and thus oxalate
absorption. We further propose that rates of bacterial oxalage
degradation are reduced in the colon of patients with enteric
hyperoxaluria, and this this is a factor leading to hyperoxaluria.

Evidence to support this hypothesis is based on our finding that
the mean rate of oxalate degradation by bacteria in 8 fecal samples
from 6 normal subjects was 2.14 ± 1.9 umoles/g/h; with a range from
4.8 to 0.1 umoles/g/h. With fecal samples from 8 JI bypass
patients, oxalate degradation rates were negligible or too low to
measure in 5 samples and rates in the other samples were 0.002,
0.004, and 0.006 umoles/g/h. Oxalate degradation rates were
estimated from measurements of $^{14}CO_2$ produced during _in vitro_
incubations of feces with ^{14}C-oxalate for 1-2 h.

The oxalate degraders we have isolated from human feces are
similar to bacteria isolated by Dawson from the rumen. They are
obligately anaerobic, gram-negative, curved rods that utilize few,
if any, substrates other than oxalate. Reasons for the apparently
lowered concentrations of these bacteria in JU bypass patients are
not yet known, but the chronic diarrheal state of these patients may
be a factor.

EFFECTS OF CLOSTRIDIUM DIFFICILE TOXIN B ON MACROMOLECULAR SYNTHESIS
IN HUMAN LUNG FIBROBLASTS AND CECAL EPITHERLIAL CELLS

C. Pothoulakie, N. Wedel, C. Franzblau and J.T. LaMont, Evans
Department of Clinical Research, Section of Gastroenterology and
Department of Biochemistry, Boston Univeristy School of Medicine,
Boston, MA 02118

C.difficile produces a potent cytotoxin, toxin B, which causes
cell rounding and disorganizes actin microfilaments in human lung
fibroblasts (IMR-90s). We carried out this study because several
other toxins exert their effect by inhibiting protein synthesis at
very low concentrations.

C. difficile toxin B was purified by the method of Sullivan et
al. Protein and DNA synthesis was measured by ^{3}H-leucine and
^{3}H-thymidine incorporation into TCA precipitates of toxin-exposed
IMR-90 fibroblasts and hamster cecal epithelial explants.

High concentrations of toxin (20 ng/ml) inhibited protein and
DNA synthesis in confluent IMR-90s after 1 and 2 hours exposure
(p 0.01). Lower doses of toxin (1 and 2 ng/ml) stimulated (p
0.01) and much lower doses had no effect on protein synthesis.
There was lack of correlation between cell rounding and alterations
in macromolecular synthesis. Similar effects were obtained with
synchronized cells. Toxin B (10 ng/ml) also decreased DNA synthesis
in hamster cecal explants after 1, 2 and 4 hours exposure (p 0.05)
without producing any morphologic alterations on the light
microscope level.

In summary, C. difficile toxin B alters macromolecular synthesis
in IMR-90 fibroblasts in a dose-dependent fashion, independently
from cell rounding. Toxin B also inhibits DNA synthesis in hamster
cecal epithelial cells.

We conclude that inhibition of macromolecular synthesis may be
an important factor in C. difficile colitis.

METHANOGENS AND TOTAL ANAEROBES IN A COLON SEGMENT ISOLATED FROM THE
NORMAL FECAL STREAM

Gray Weaver M.D., Meyer J. Wolin, Ph.D., and Terry L. Miller Ph.D.
The Mary Imogene Bassett Hospital, Cooperstown, NY and the New York
State Health Department, Albany, NY.

The bacterial composition of samples taken from the remaining
colon of an 80 year old women were studied. Samples were taken 14
months after the patient had a left hemicolectomy with end colostomy
and mucous fistula for near obstruction in the mid sigmoid colon of
unknown etiology. Fecal material from the colostomy bag (draining
the right colon and transverse colon) and from the rectum (mucous
fistula) were studied. The concentration (per g dry weight) ot
total anaerobes of the brown liquid from the colostomy bat and the
creamy white paste of the rectal sample were 5.9×10^{11} and $1.2 \times
10^{10}$, respectively. Methanogens were less than 1×10^{4} in the
colostomy sample and = or than 5×10^{7} per g dry weight in the
rectal sample. The predominant methanogens of the rectal sample
were isolated and identified as Methanobrevibacter smithii. The
results indicate that a normal anaerobic bacterial community and
anaerobic fermentation was supported by non-dietary substrates in
the portion of the lower bowel that was disconnected from the upper
gastronintestinal tract and remaining large bowel.

PILI MEDIATE THE ABILITY OF <u>ESCHERICHIA COLI</u> (RDEC-1) BACTERIA TO ADHERS, BUT NOT TO PERSIST, ON RABBIT ILEAL LYMPHOID FOLLICLE EPITHELIUM

Lindsey R. Inman and J. Robert Cantey, Veterans Administration Medical Center, Charleston, SC, 29403.

The rabbit enteropathogenic <u>Escherichia coli</u> (strain RDEC-1) adheres to M cells in the lymphoid follicle epithelium of rabbits within hours and to gut epithelium three days postinoculation. An 85 Md plasmid mediates the expression of pili associated with the adherence of the bacterium to ileal brush border preparations.

We obtained for use in this study two nonpathogenic <u>Shigella flexneri</u> 2a strains, SHD15 which contained the 85 Md plasmid and expressed RDEC-1 pili, and a control strain, ShD12. Cryostat sections of Peyer's patch tissue taken at two, four, six, and 12 hours post-orogastric-inoculation with 2×10^{10} ShD15, ShD12, or RDEC-1 bacteria, when stained with specific FITC labelled antibody, revealed that the ShD12 strain did not adhere to the lymphoid follicle epithelium. The ShD15 strain was seen adhering in large numbers at two and four hours, less at six hours and was not demonstrable by 12 hours postinoculation. The RDEC-1 strain adhered in increasing numbers through 12 hours.

Lymphoid follicle tissue from rabbits challenged with ShD12 strain demonstrated normal epithelium with no associated bacteria when examined by transmission electronmicroscopy. Two hours post-innoculation with the ShD15 strain intralumenal and intraepithelial bacteria were seen, by six hours an acute inflammatory response, characterized by prominent intralumenal and intraepithelial polymorphonuclear leukocytes with erosion of the lymphoid follicle epithelium, had occurred. Minimal or no inflammation occurred with RDEC-1 lymphoid follicle adherence.

RDEC-1 pili mediate initial adherence to lymphoid follicle epithelium but other factors, which the ShD15 strain lacks, make it possible for the RDEC-1 strain to persist on the follicle without precipitating an acute inflammatory response.

ASSOCIATION OF GERMFREE MICE WITH CONVENTIONAL HAMSTER FLORA

K.H. Wilson, J.N. Sheagren and R. Freter, Infectious Disease Section and Medical Service, Veterans Administration Medical Center and Departments of Medicine and Microbiology and Immunology, University of Michigan Medical School, Ann Arbor, MI.

The Syrian hamster, the major animal model for Clostridium difficile colitis, is not available in the germfree state. The works of Raibaud et al, Hazenberg et al and Ducluzeau et al suggest that the colonic flora of one species may be studied in gnotobiotic animals of another species. To test the feasibility of studying the hamster's cecal flora in a gnotobiotic model, we associated germfree Swiss mice with C. difficile (strain 49-A) and a streptomycin resistant strain of E. coli (C-25). Either a conventional mouse or a conventional hamster was then paced into the isolators with the diassociated mice. Three weeks later, animals were sacrificed, ceca weighed and C. difficile and E. coli population sizes quantitated on selective media.

	Cecal Size (% body weight)	Log^{10} CFU Per Cecum C. difficile	E. Coli
Diassociated (N=6)	5.2 $\pm$ .2% ($\pm$ s.e.m.)	7.6 $\pm$ .1	10.4 $\pm$ .1
Mouse Associated (N=10)	2.3 $\pm$ .1%	2.5	3.0 $\pm$ .9
Hamster Associated (N-12)	2.6 $\pm$ .1%	2.5 to 2.9	2.6 $\pm$ .7

Conventional hamster flora is able to assume in mice complex functions such as reduction of cecal size and suppression of both coliform bacteria and C. difficile. In addition, Gram stains of cecal contents from hamster-associated mice were indistinguishable from stains of hamster cecal contents.

Abstract # 15

SPIROCHETES OF THE RAT GASTROINTESTINAL TRACT

COWLEY H. M. AND HILL R.R.H.
Department of Infectious Diseases, University of Witwatersand,
1, Jan Smuts Avenue, Braafontein, Johannesburg, 2001, South Africa.

A survey of the rat gastrointestinal tract by electron microscopy, revealed the presence of four dominant spirochete morphotypes. These bacteria were confined to the large bowel and were specifically associated with either the mucosal epithelial surface or with the lumen contents. Only one type was seen in both habitats. Successful _in vitro_ culture of strains belonging to all four morphotypes, revealed little variation in their fastidious nutritional requirements and biochemical reactions. The anaerobic growth conditions, serum or short chain fatty acid requirements and the ability to digest mucin all indicate that these organisms are adapted to their _in vivo_ habitat, although their precise role in the gastrointestinal ecosystem has yet to be elucidated.

Abstract # 16

COLONIZATION RESISTANCE OF THE GASTROINTESTINAL TRACT - A POTENTIAL

LIGNAN PRODUCTION BY FAECAL FLORA

S.P. BORRIELLO AND K.D.R. SETCHELL. Clinical Research Centre,
Watford Road, Harrow, Middlesex, HA1 3UJ.

Until the recent description of enterolactone and enterodiol as
the major lignans present in the urine of humans, they had only been
found in higher plants. Initial interest in these compounds was
stimulated by the demonstration of a cyclic excretion pattern during
the menstrual cycle, which was suggestive of a physiological role.
Recent work has shown that synthetic enterolactone can significantly
depress oestrogen-stimulated rat uterine cytosol RNA synthesis and
that it is cytotoxic to human lymphoid cells. In addition many
lignans are effective against animal tumours, and some have been
subjected to clinical trials. This led to the speculation that they
may protect against cancer in man. It has recently been shown that
lignan excretion is lower in women who have breast cancer than
healthy controls.

We have shown that excretion of these compounds is depressed in
subjects receiving antibiotics, which was fairly good indirect
evidence that the gastrointestinal flora probably played a part in
the production of these compounds in man. We have now shown that
these compounds can be formed by the faecal flora in vitro and shown
that enterolactone is the oxidized product of enterodiol. This
metabolic step is carried out by facultative bacteria. By
co-incubation of faecal flora with linseeds and with
secoisolariciresinol, a constituent of linseed, we have also been
able to produce both lignans. This reaction is also carried out by
facultative bacteria. In a further study we produced enterolactone
from matairesinol, a more abundant plant lignan than
secoisolariciresinol, after incubation under either aerobic or
anaerobic conditions. There appear to be a number of similar
pathways operative that can produce enterolactone and enterodiol
depending on the major dietary precursor ingested.

Abstract # 17

COLONIZATION RESISTANCE OF THE GASTROINTESTINAL TRACT - A POTENTIAL
IN VITRO METHOD FOR THE DETERMINATION OF SUSCEPTIBILITY TO INFECTION
WITH C.DIFFICILE

S.P. BORRIELLO AND FIONA BARCLAY, CLINICAL RESEARCH CENTRE, WATFORD
ROAD, HARROW, HA1 3UJ.

The administration of antimicrobials may result in disruption of
the normal gut flora and can pre-dispose to C.difficile infection.
To show the importance of the normal gut flora in preventing the
establishment of C.difficile in vivo we have developed an in vitro
test system based on growth in faecal emulsions. Cytotoxigenic
C.difficile were added to dilutions of stool specimens from 18
healthy adults and 30 patients with antibiotic-associated diarrhoea
(AAD) who were negative for C.difficile and its cytotoxin. These
were incubated anaerobically for 72 h and both total and spore
counts performed at 24 h intervals. Toxin and pH levels were also
estimated. In parallel, emulsions prepared from normal stools were
sterilized by autoclaving or centrifugation and filtration. Growth
of C.difficile was inhibited when in the presence of the faecal
flora of healthy volunteers. Sterile faecal emulsions or filtrates
of these stool samples were no longer inhibitory, showing the
importance of viable bacteria. Eight of the AAD stools failed to
inhibit C.difficile. One of these patients subsequently became
colonized. The filtrates of 13 of the 22 inhibitory AAD stools were
shown to be inhibitory which probably reflects inhibitory faecal
levels of the offending antibiotic. Stools found to be positive for
C.difficile on original culture were also tested for their ability
to inhibit the organism. In these cases the levels of indigenous
C.difficile were measured. No growth inhibition could be
demonstrated. These observations highlight the importance of a
normal gut flora in prevention of disease and indicate that it may

be possible to identify those patients at risk by use of an <u>in vitro</u> test system. This system has now been used to look at colonization resistance potential in healthy infants and healthy adults of different age groups. Preliminary results on our studies to find an indirect chemical marker that correlates with this bio-assay will also be presented.

Abstract # 18

CORRELATION OF HYPOPROTHROMBINEMIA WITH SUPPRESSION OF MENAQUINONE
PRODUCING INTESTINAL MICROFLORA

K. RAMOTAR, J. CONLY, E. BOW, A. RONALD AND T.J. LOUIE, UNIVERSITY
OF MANITOBA, WINNIPEG, CANADA.

One hundred and eight patients randomized to receive either
moxalactam plus ticarcillin (M/T) or tobramycin plus ticarcillin
(T/T) in a prospective clinical trial of empiric antimicrobial
therapy for febrile neutropenic episodes in cancer patients had
serial prothrombin times (PT) evaluated to determine the incidence
of hypoprothrombinemia (HPT). HPT was defined as a PT 2 seconds
beyond control. Thirty of 54 patients in the M/T and 13/54 patients
in the T/T group had HPT (p .01). Ten of 54 patients in the M/T
and 3/54 patients in the T/T groups had clinically significant
bleeding episodes. The patients in each group were comparable with
respect to age, sex, diagnosis, chemotherapy, infection category,
outcome and initial granulocyte count. Serial quantitative faecal
cultures of M/T patients revealed that facultatively anaerobic
Gram-negative bacilli, primarily E.coli, and obligate anaerobic
Gram-negative bacilli, primarily Bacteroides spp., were reduced to
counts of 10^3CFU/gram wet weight of stool. In contrast, E.coli
and Bacteroides spp. persisted in the majority of T/T patients.
Using preparative and analytical TLC, menaquinone profiles were
examined in selected faecal organisms including E.coli (5),
B.fragilis (5), B.ovatus (6), B.distasonis (6), B.thetaiotamicron
(2), B.vulgatus (5), B.bivius (2), B.disiens (1), Fusobacterium spp.
(4), Peptococcus spp. (4), Peptostreptococcus spp. (5),
Propionibacteria spp. (9), Bifedobacterium spp. (4), Eubacterium
spp. (4), Lactobacillus Spp. (5), C.perfringens (5) and Clostridium
spp. (6). Menaquinones were produced by all strains of E.coli

(MK-8), all Bacteroides spp. (MK-9, 10, 11, 12), 6 of 9
Propionibacterium spp. (MK-n) and 2 of 4 Eubacterium spp. (MK-n).
These data suggest that intestinal microflora may be an important
source of vitamin K in patients who have a reduced intake of
exogenous vitamin K_1.

Abstract # 19

RABBIT ENTEROTOXAEMIA: CHARACTERISTICS OF CLOSTRIDIUM SPIROFORME
AND ITS TOXIN

R.J. CARMAN[+], S.P. BORRIELLO[*] AND A.B. PRICE[*]
[+] Charing Cross Hospital Medical School, St.Dunstan's Road, London
W6 8RP, England and [*] Clinical Research Centre, Watford Road,
Harrow, Middlesex HA6 3UJ, England.

Clostridium spiroforme is the cause of diarrhoea in both natural
and antibiotic associated enterotoxaemia of rabbits. In vitro the
organism produces a toxin which can be neutralized by C.perfringens
Type E iota antitoxin. A similar toxin can be shown to be present
in the caeca of diarrhoeic rabbits. The toxin was almost invariably
found in all those animals harbouring C.spiroforme. If newly weaned
or clindamycin treated rabbits are housed in isolators they remain
free of diarrhoea until orally challenged with C.spiroforme. In
mature animals both antibiotic and organism are necessary to produce
the disease. Neither alone is sufficient. Changes in the
alimentary tract ecology are thought to be the main factors
predisposing rabbits to the condition.

C.spiroforme toxin produced in vitro is biologically active only
when it is pretreated with trypsin. Following heating to 56°C for
30 minutes activity is lost. It is lethal for mice when injected
intraperitoneally. Hind limb paralysis usually precedes death.
Intradermal challenge of depilated guinea pigs produces a
characteristic necrotic lesion. The toxin is cytotoxic to Vero,
MRC5 and HeLa cells in tissue culture. Fluid accumulation,
indicating enterotoxic activity, can be seen in the infant mouse
assay and the ligated rabbit ileal loop. In the latter, the degree
of inflammation and villus degeneration is proportional to the
relative amount of fluid accumulation. All these activities can be
neutralized by C.perfringens Type E iota antitoxin.

R.J.C. receives a grant from Ralston Purina Europe S.A.